To my Mom:

Who gave me the world.

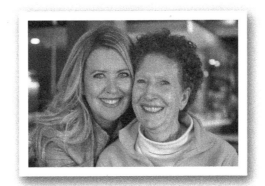

FROM THE

Sticky Fingers cooking™

SCHOOL

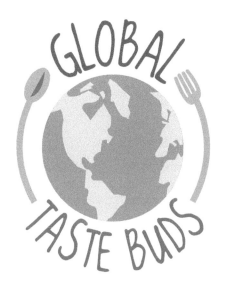

The First Cookbook
GLOBAL TASTE BUDS
Cook and Eat Your Way
Around the World!

"To travel is to live."
- Hans Christian Andersen

"You have to taste a culture to understand it."
- Deborah Cater

**"I love everything we cook with
Sticky Fingers!"**
- Young Chef Gideon

"I love it SO MUCH, it's freaking me out!"

- Lexi, age 8 (after tasting the very delicious Zany Stuffed Spring Rolls + Crispy Crazy Potstickers she just made) page 39

"This is so great! BETTER than Pizza!"

- Monica, age 7 (after tasting her India's Turnip Tikka Masala + Street-Style Hakka Noodles + Classic Indian Sweet Yogurt Lassi) page 10

the Sticky Fingers Cooking School

Sticky Fingers Cooking is an acclaimed mobile and online children's cooking school providing inspiring "hands-on" cooking classes to over 50,000 students since 2011. We recognize the value of fostering curiosity, independence, confidence, and development of essential, lifelong cooking skills through interactive and engaging culinary experiences.

We whisk together a sense of fun within all of our specially-developed, kid-friendly curriculum and in our over 800 proprietary recipes designed to expand children's skills and palates. We combine and connect our love of culinary arts with nutritional information, safe cooking skills, language, geography, math, science, and food history to help inspire and ignite a lifetime love of healthy cooking and adventurous eating that children relish.

"These doughnut holes are infinity percent vitamin C delicious!"

- Tae-ji, age 8 (loving the Italian Orange Carrot Polenta Zeppole + Italian Cocoa Orange Lattes he just had a blast making) page 43

"I can't believe there is corn in our Mac 'n Cheese! Yum!"

Enthusiastic Young Chef (savoring her just-made Corny Veggie Mac 'n Cheese Cups + Crispy Veggie Streusel Crust + Classic Pink Lemonade) page 83

Here's a quick view of all the wonderful places the delicious
Global Taste Buds recipes come from!

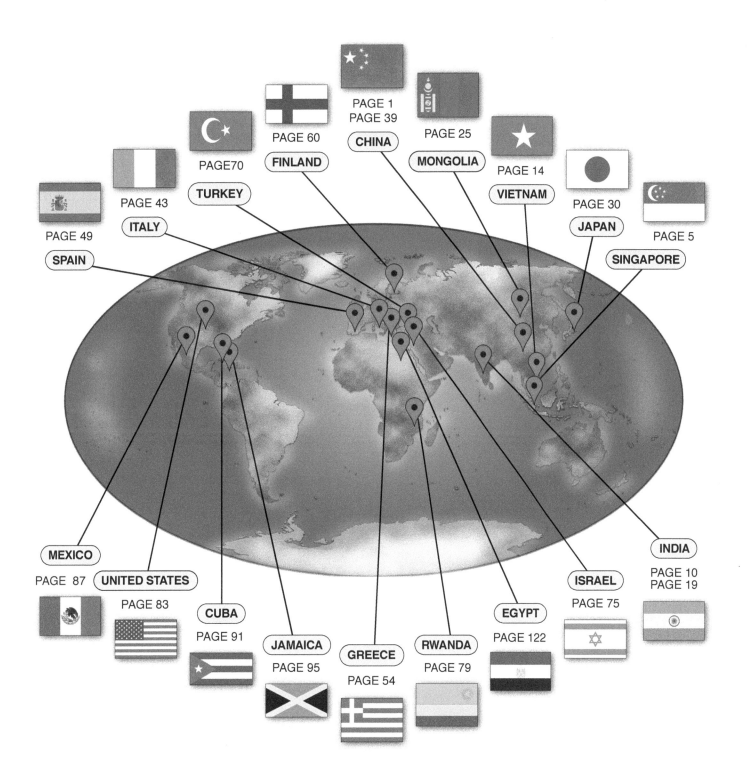

How much tasty fun will you have exploring the World as you get to make and
enjoy so many delicious recipes kids around the World also love?

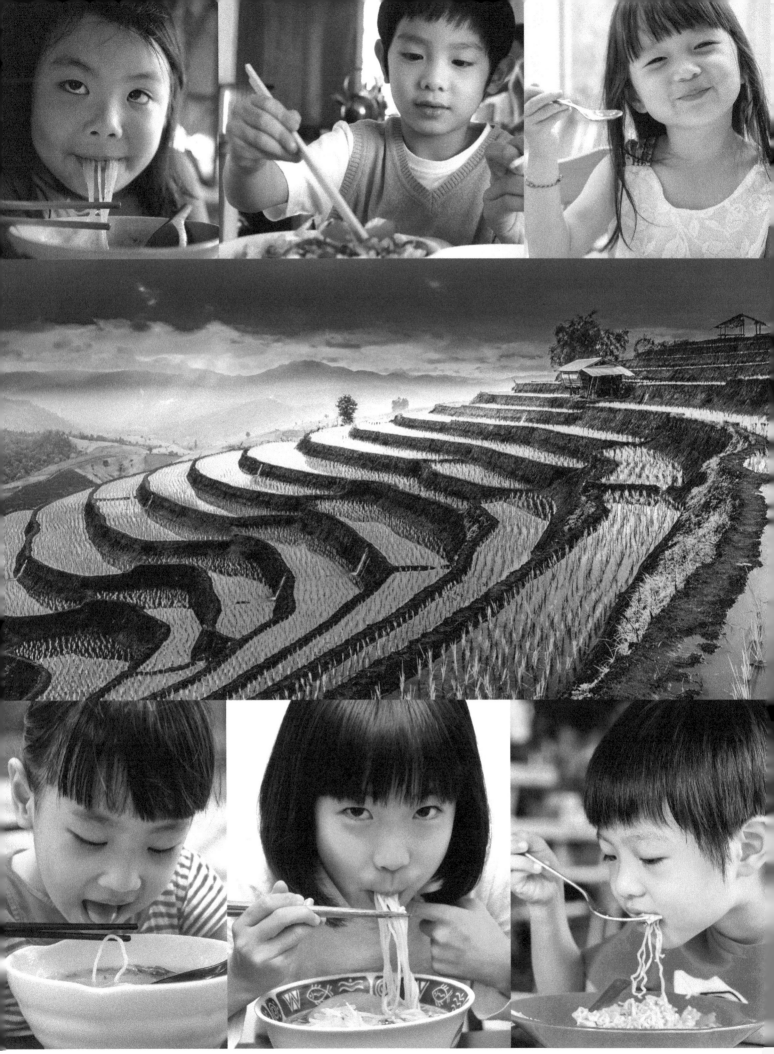

STREET FOOD RECIPES FROM ASIA

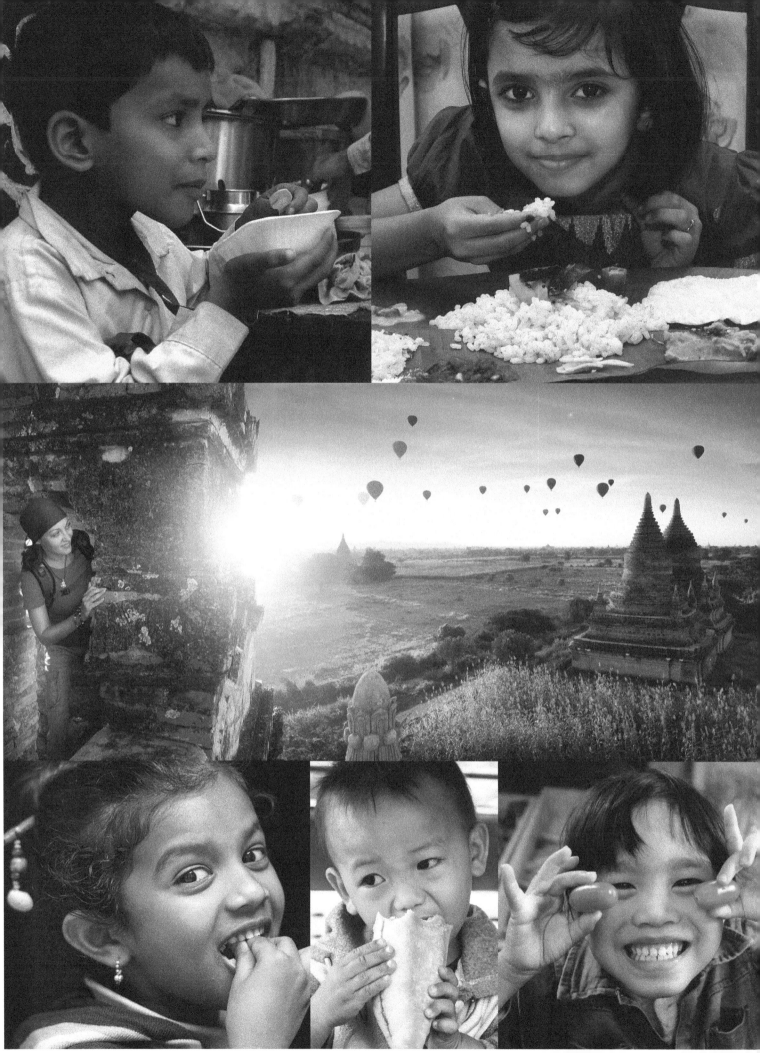

MORE RECIPES
FROM ASIA

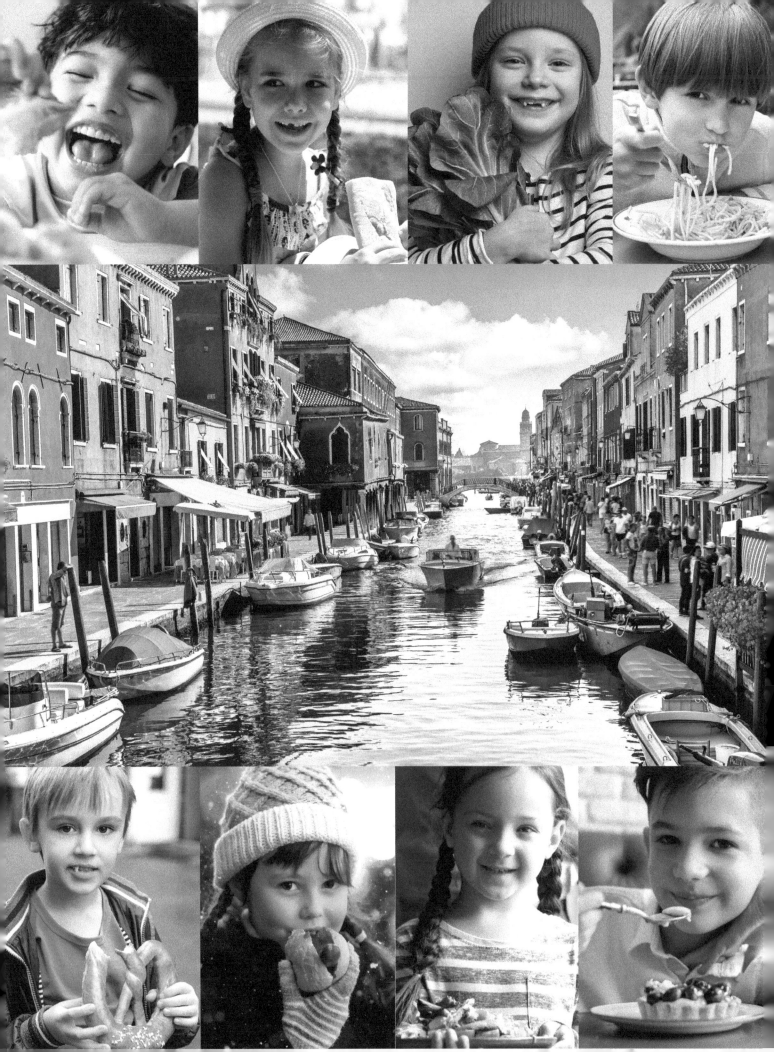

RECIPES FROM EUROPE

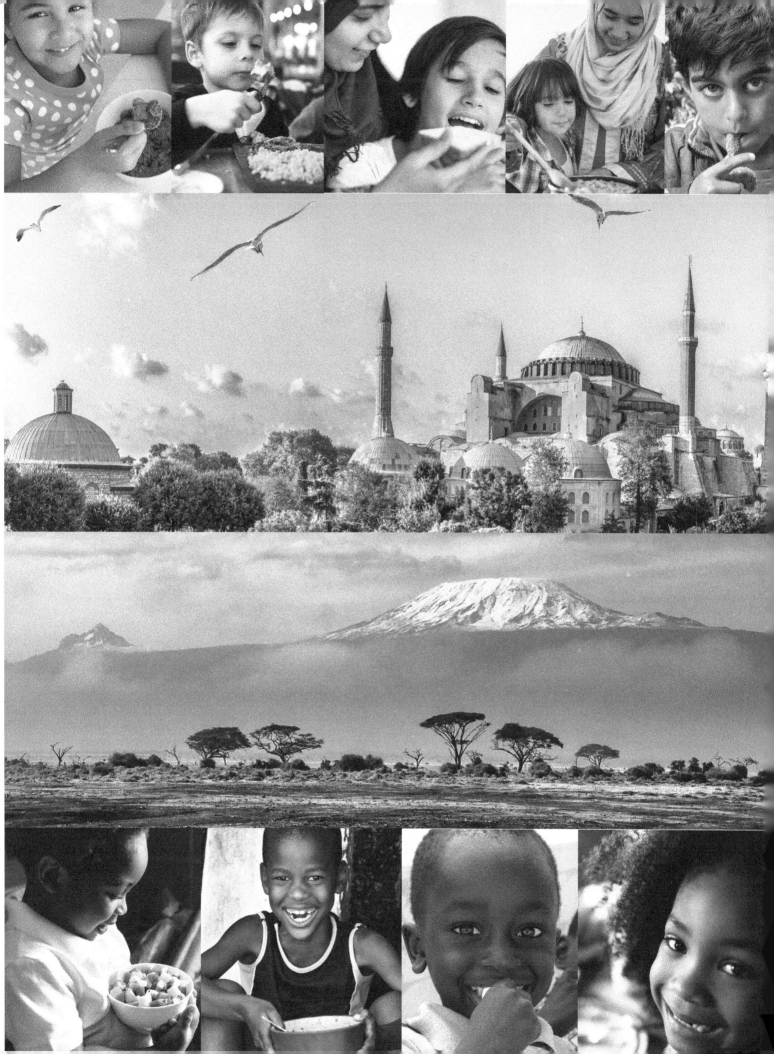

RECIPES FROM THE MIDDLE EAST & AFRICA

EGYPT

TURKEY

ISRAEL

RWANDA

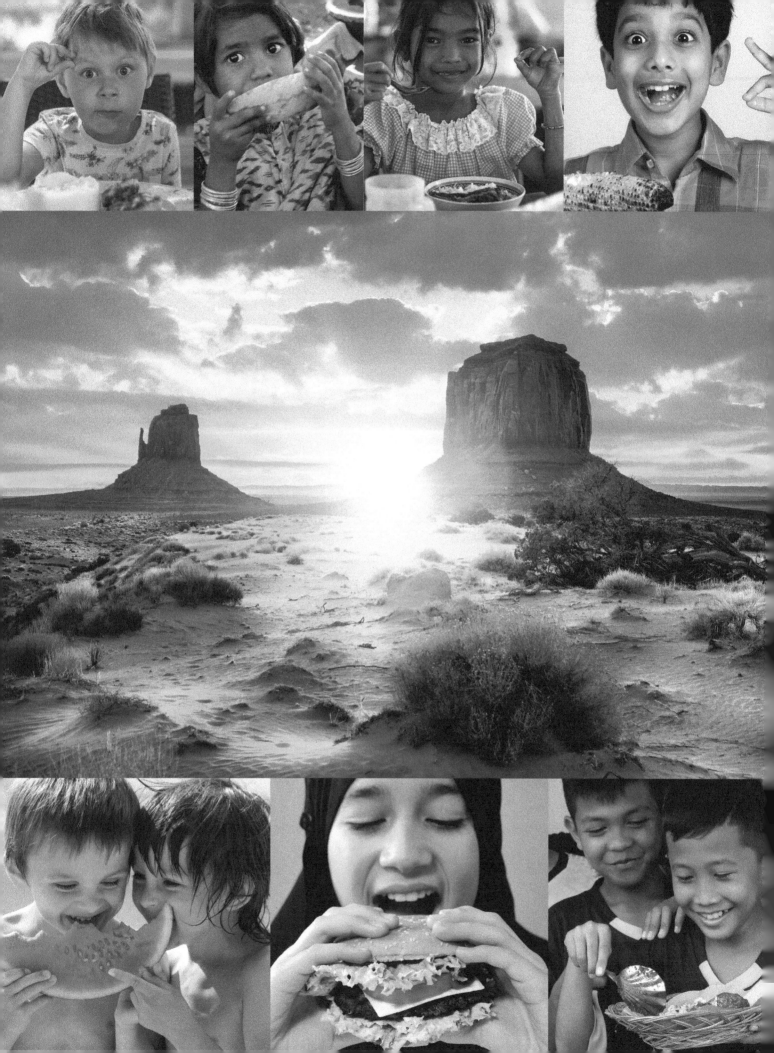

RECIPES FROM THE AMERICAS

UNITED STATES

MEXICO

CUBA

JAMAICA

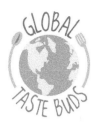

INTRODUCTION

Welcome to Sticky Fingers Cooking's Global Taste Buds Cookbook!

Global Taste Buds had to be our first Sticky Fingers Cooking cookbook for so many reasons.

Food is one of the most interesting, accessible and delicious ways to get to know a culture from the inside. Being exposed to new cultures lays a strong foundation for children to become citizens of the world—to develop a profound sense of understanding and respect for other people, to foster the know-how to coexist with each other peacefully, to cultivate the self-reliance needed to successfully navigate new places and situations.

Like travel, cooking opens your world to new adventure and opportunity with each step you take —the chance to say yes to something new.

If you really want to learn about a country, eat and cook the way its people do. Cooking opens the door to other cultures in a way that nothing else can, like you have been invited to pull up a chair and sit at the family table for a special feast. We can fold the map and travel across geography, history, time and space by preparing and eating foods our fellow humans enjoy around the world.

Do you know a child who only eats cheese pizza or chicken fingers? Not every kid dives spoon first into a bowl of Tikka Masala or takes a bite of sushi for the first time without hesitation. But they will if they cook it!

When you present a new ingredient to a kid, and they are in charge of learning what it is and how to prepare it, something magical happens—they willingly venture out of their culinary comfort zone and challenge themselves in new ways. The confidence they gain is priceless.

I never tire of seeing this miraculous transformation unfold, and it has happened in each and every class ever taught at Sticky Fingers Cooking. Cooking encourages exploration and makes kids want to try new foods without our prompting. If they make it, they'll eat it!

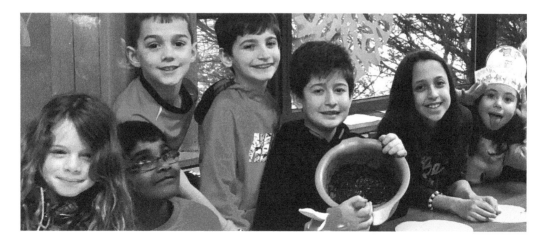

I'm Erin Fletter—Food Geek-in-Chief, recipe developer, mom, wife, and avid (some would rightly say fanatical) traveler!

My first journey to a new country was Mexico when I was 6 years old. My parents and I took a train from Mexicali where we bought a bag of freshly baked, crusty bolillos rolls for the journey down the Sonoran coast to Mazatlán. The we hopped on a ferry and ended up in Cabo San Lucas where we ate rich lobster tacos and crisp churros from roadside stands under the warm sun. It was the most exciting thing in my life and forever changed the way I see the world. Food and travel have played a fundamental role in my own life.

As a teen, I was lucky enough to have the world's most adventurous mom. We would spin the globe on my desk and pick one place to visit every year, often for a month or two at a time, with just our backpacks and each other. Our travels were full of incredible discoveries exploring and learning about many other countries, people and cultures around the world.

We journeyed to every continent except Antarctica, exploring and learning along the way.
It shaped who I am, and how I see the world. Food is a necessity for all life. Cooking is an elemental and extraordinary life skill that connects us all.

Travel can have a far-reaching impact on kids. Kids who travel are more likely to have higher independence, self-esteem, confidence, adaptability and sensitivity. Yet, impactful travel doesn't necessarily have to be jaunts around the globe, exploring new worlds. Just by cooking and eating global foods, you will kickstart your children's curiosity and love for the world around them.

I am so excited that you have found our collection of global recipesw—I hope you are just as excited to begin your cooking adventure and travel the globe right from your own kitchen!
Come cook up some fun and taste the world with us!

- Erin Fletter, Food-Geek-In-Chief, Co-Founder
Sticky Fingers Cooking

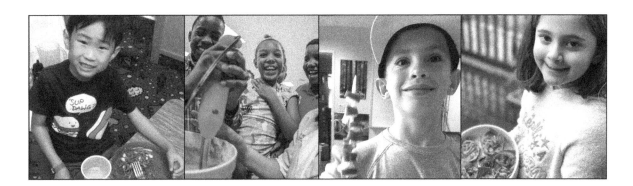

HOW TO USE THE COOKBOOK

In this delicious and adventurous cookbook, young chefs and their families can cook 20 full-meal recipes from countries all around the world. You and your young chefs will cook up and gobble up tasty, healthy cuisine from the Americas, Europe, Africa, the Middle East, and Asia while exploring customs, geography, food history, activities, people, and languages of these diverse cultures.

Cooking with kids is not precise and there is always room for flexibility and creativity. The simple miracle of cooking with your kids: If they make it, they want to eat it. We know that anyone can cook. Everyone should cook. We know that kids make the best cooks because they always naturally make it fun!

The recipes in this cookbook are all flexible and fun, written with small hands and young, creative kids in mind. If you don't have a specific ingredient, please don't fret! Call on your imagination and find something that you can use in its place. Find adventure in the kitchen and even, at times, adventure in a half empty refrigerator. Make things colorful.

Here are some quick and super easy ingredient substitution examples:

★ Use diced apples in place of blueberries

★ Replace carrots with the zucchini in a recipe

★ Add all the colorful bell peppers to your recipes

★ Experiment with using purple cauliflower vs. white cauliflower

One of the best things about cooking is that it can transport us to faraway places we've only dreamed of, while also exposing us to new foods and connecting us to our diverse and delicious, global cultures. When you flip through this book you will notice that our recipes are much, much more than stand-alone recipes. These recipes are a world in and of themselves. These are 20 complete meals and unique experiences and activities meant to transport you and your family to new adventures where you will learn about food history, cultures, nutrition, and language, with even a few bad food jokes—haha—sprinkled in.

We encourage your family to pick and choose from these recipes… Mix and match! The most important recipes in this book are those that become your favorites to prepare and the most relevant to you and your family. Explore. Break the "rules."

You will also find kitchen vocabulary words and cooking vernacular sprinkled into our recipes as well as "how-to" cooking techniques in many of the recipes. This is to reinforce proper cooking techniques throughout the book for kids to build on mastering their own cooking skills in the kitchen.

You may notice that our recipes do not contain much, if any, meat products. Sticky Fingers Cooking started as a mobile cooking school and we did not see the need to complicate things with bringing in meat, poultry or seafood to our classes. Imagine a kindergartener cutting up chicken in a classroom. No thank you! While we create and prepare mostly plant-based recipes with kids, we do not highlight it, and most of our families and students do not even realize our recipes are actually plant based.

We are an inclusive school and cook with kids with a myriad of food allergies, celiac, Type 1 diabetes and we also often have kosher food cooking classes as well. We believe that we can ALL be eating more be eating more plant-based foods. That doesn't hurt anyone! We encourage your family to freely add in your favorite protein, meats, seafoods according to your family's preference. Please do! We believe in good food no matter what! We eat everything ourselves… No judgments! Of course, we hope to expand your famiy's horizons and palates a bit in the process.

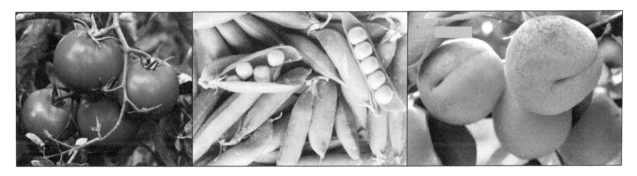

Fresh ingredients and where our food comes from is a truly essential focus of Sticky Fingers Cooking. You may notice that we have many images of fresh foods, and do not include photos of what the end result of each recipe 'should' be. This is entirely intentional. I, myself, get intimidated by beautiful photos of what a dish 'should' look like in cookbooks and can become vastly disappointed in myself when it looks (crazy) different. That fear of "failure" keeps people from trying. From exploring. From getting curious. Why would we subject our children to this nonsense? It's like a kid taking an art class and the teacher says, "here kids, this is the Mona Lisa, here are some paints. Go do that."

We have seen extremely funky, extremely creative and extremely delicious recipe creations over the years from the 50,000+ students in our cooking classes. We are thrilled to say that we have a 100% approval rating from our students who are proud of their own unique food stylings. We encourage you all to embrace all of the ways your family interacts with and interprets our recipes without fear… without rules.

If you only take one thing away from this cookbook, we hope it's the most important morsel: We want your family to enjoy the pleasures of cooking and eating with people you love most!

LETTUCE GET OUR EQUIPMENT ORGANIZED

- [ ] A chef's knife (more on that later)
- [ ] Cutting board
- [ ] Measuring cups & spoons
- [ ] Pots & pans
- [ ] Spatula
- [ ] Whisk
- [ ] Pastry brush
- [ ] Large stirring spoon
- [ ] Oven mitts
- [ ] Glass baking dish
- [ ] Grater
- [ ] Metal muffin pan
- [ ] Metal baking sheet
- [ ] Colander
- [ ] Can opener

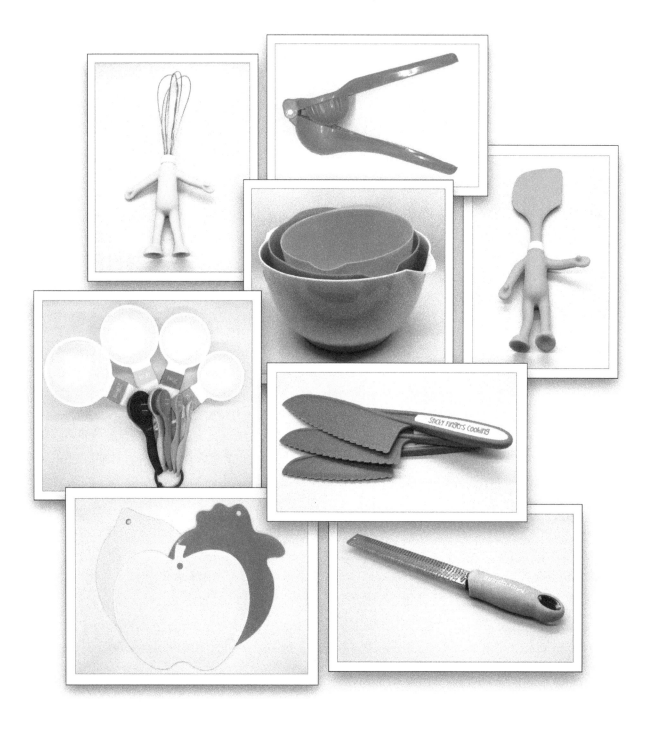

K'NIFTY KNIFE SKILLS

Let's get straight to the point! We like to use small, plastic lettuce knives when cooking with kids. They have "teeth" to cut through foods but are not sharp. Here are some simple tips on getting started:

DUH! This may sound silly and obvious, but when picking up a knife, it is important to notice which side is dull and which side is sharp. Always walk with the knife tip down.

MASTERY: For the best control, your hand should be all the way at the top of the handle where the blade and handle meet. You will be a master chef in no time!

STABLE TABLE: Make sure you have a stable, clear surface to cut on, such as a cutting mat or board. If your board is slipping around, place a piece of damp paper towel underneath to keep it from moving.

PREP: It may sometimes be necessary for your parents to partly prepare or cut some foods down for you so they are at a stage where you can handle them safely and confidently yourself.

LAY DOWN FLAT: Make sure that the food being cut has a flat surface or the most stable surface is face down on the chopping board, so it is stable while being cut and not all wobbly.

HURRY UP AND S-L-O-W DOWN: Developing knife skills takes practice, so take your time to find your own pace and rhythm before adding speed.

SOFT: Start practicing with very soft foods like bananas, zucchini, cucumbers, and strawberries.

SAW: Practice making a sawing motion: "back and forth…back and forth."

THE BEAR CLAW (GROWL!): This Is easy to remember. It is the shape your hand should be making while you do it! Curl all the fingers and the thumb of your non-knife hand like you're imitating an angry bear (growl!). Keep this hand shape and press the tips of your fingers (nails) to grip against the food. Now make a sawing motion: *"back and forth…back and forth."* This ensures that your fingertips (or claws) are tucked out of the way and will not get caught by the knife. The "bear claw" is the best method to use when food needs to be cut into slices or diced up.

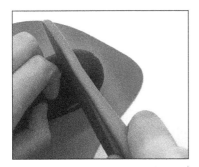 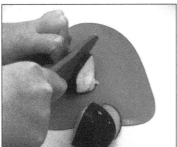 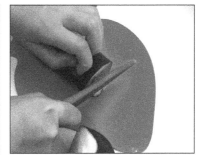

THE BRIDGE + TUNNEL (ZOOM, ZOOM!): Create a bridge over the food with your hand. The fingers should be on one side and the thumb should be on the other. Hold the food between your fingers and thumb. That's your bridge. The knife then goes underneath your "bridge" and into the "tunnel" so your hand is completely safe and cannot be cut. Now make a sawing motion: "back and forth…back and forth." To help remember this method, think of the knife as a car which goes under the bridge and through the tunnel. ZOOM-ZOOM! This method is great for cutting circular items into halves and quarters: e.g., tomatoes, apples, eggplant, oranges.

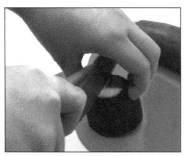 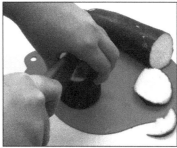 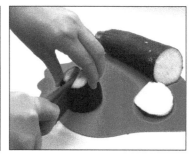

PLANK (SAW, SAW, SPLAT!): After gently sawing back and forth to start a little cut in the food, place your free hand (the one not holding the knife) on top of the dull part of the knife to push down and add extra pressure to cut through the food. Saw, saw, SPLAT! This method is great for cutting soft items into halves, quarters, and cubes: e.g., bananas, tofu, zucchini, cheese.

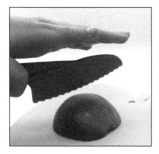 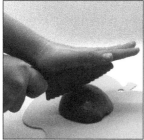 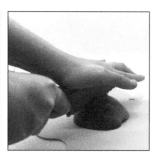 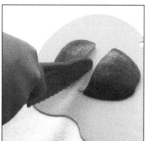

PEELING: Always peel away from yourself while using a peeler. With long foods such as carrots, hold one end, peel from the middle away from yourself, and then hold the peeled end and repeat the same process.

GRATING: Remember, you do not have to grate every bit of the food. It is best to leave a small chunk at the end to hang on to. This means that your fingers are never pressed against the grater.

SCISSORS: Kitchen scissors can sometimes be a useful alternative to a knife, especially if you have small hands. Scissors are good for snipping herbs and spring onions–even pepper slices!

CLEANING UP TIPS and TRICKS FOR PARENTS

**"I love cleaning up messes I didn't make.
So I became a parent."**
- Said no parent EVER

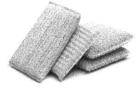

FOR PARENTS:

Children love to cook. Children love to make a mess... but cleaning? Perhaps, not as much. We are here to help! Studies show that giving children household chores at an early age helps to build a lasting sense of mastery, responsibility, and self-reliance. Kids who started doing chores early, as young as toddlers, are more likely to have academic success, to have good relationships with friends and family, and eventually success in their careers, when compared with those who didn't have chores as young kids.

Just as cooking is an essential life skill, so is cleaning. Here are a few ways to incorporate and encourage cleaning for the youngest members of your family.

★ **Cleaning is not punishment!** How many times as a child were you asked to clean something as a form of punishment? Too many times to count. If you are negative and talk to your kids about being messy and having to clean as a punitive activity in a grumpy manner, they will be grumpy and negative right back. A better message to offer children is that cleaning is not a punishment but rather simply a way of life, not a big deal. Cleaning is something that must be done, and it's a part of cooperating and being part of a family. A fabulous motivator for children is once things are tidy, we are ready to create again!

★ **Talk about cleaning & health:** Help your child connect the dots on why a messy home isn't a great thing. Just as we clean our hands before we eat, we need to keep our kitchen clean before and after cooking. It is helpful to explain how germs travel, how bugs or rodents can be attracted to dirty dishes or crumbs, and if our food is left out, unrefrigerated, it can spoil and become unsafe to eat. We want to keep ourselves, our family, and our home healthy and safe.

★ **Give choices:** This is a Sticky Fingers Cooking FAVORITE. Being in control of yourself and making decisions is something that is especially important to kids, as most of their life is being dictated by others. The aspect of cleaning is no different. There is always a plethora of tasks in need of help every day, so why not give your children some options in the process? When children have choices and are able to use their voice, they feel independent, in control, and important. Remember: Only give two choices and make sure that you are *comfortable with either outcome.*

1. Do you want to set the table before dinner or clear the dishes after dinner?

2. Do you want to wipe off the counters or sweep the floor?

3. Do you prefer putting away the food or emptying the trash can?

4. Would you like to unload the clean dishes or wipe down the sink?

5. Would you like to wash the dishes or load them into the dishwasher? (Sticky Fingers Tip: Kids LOVE water and will be over-the-moon to wash dishes!)

6. What do you see that needs cleaning?

7. What will you choose to do to help?

★ **Fast + fun cleaning together:** Rather than asking everyone to clean separately, do it together. Teamwork makes the dream work! Remind your family that the faster everyone cleans up, the more time can be spent playing games, having fun, cooking, and relaxing.

Other Helpful Tips:

• *Establish cleaning times: After school, before school, before dinner, or after dinner. Giving children a clear routine makes them feel safe, secure, and loved.*

• *Come up with a fun name like TEAM CLEAN, SUPER CLEANERS, or CLEAN CLUB.*

• *Set 10 minutes on the clock.*

• *Play your favorite music.*

• *Everyone does their chosen cleaning job.*

• *Parents, kids, and siblings can "race" each other in clean up jobs.*

• *After 10 minutes, you may be surprised by how much you all accomplished together!*

★ **Keep it bite-sized and reward:**

• *Cleaning is ever-present and can feel overwhelming. Identify just one or two small cleaning tasks and get them done. Celebrate when this is accomplished. It is a great feeling when you get something completed, and children will see and experience that sense of joy.*

• *If there is a playdate, a movie, or a fun game that is scheduled for later that day, make that the reward. As soon as we TEAM CLEAN, we can move on with our other activities!*

• *Always remember to say "thank you" to each other and your kids. Your kids may even start noticing when you clean something on your own and say "thank you" out of the blue! It is important to lead by example. Our children are watching and listening with those perky ears!*

Remember: You're not being mean by having your children help. It establishes important, valuable routines that give children purpose. Their self-confidence will rise with every helpful effort, and that is what Sticky Fingers Cooking calls a WIN-WIN!

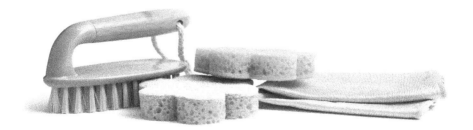

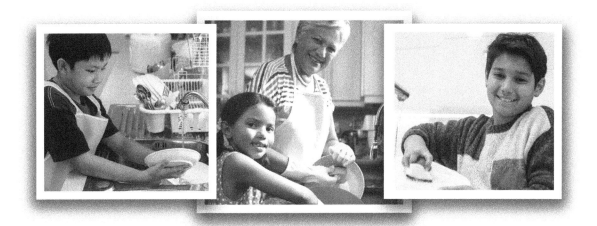

CLEANING UP TIPS and TRICKS FOR KIDS

FOR ALL STICKY FINGERS CHEFS-IN-TRAINING:

We know you love to cook! We know cleaning is a part of cooking, and sometimes that task can be challenging and not the super-duper fun part. Here are some quick tips for you, our wonderful and creative chefs:

★ **Clean as you go.** This really does make a huge difference! It is easier to clean smaller messes than larger ones.

★ **Prep stations are super fun and help keep you organized!** (And it is totally cool to pretend or imagine that you are in a restaurant and a chef!)

★ **If you are following a recipe,** it is helpful to have the book or tablet in front of you and your cook station so you can follow along easily.

★ **It is OK to ask an adult for help,** but try your hardest first. Parents love to see you succeed!

★ **If things get a little (or a lot) messy, don't panic!** Rule number one is never panic. Just take a deep breath and begin to clean or wipe up what spilled.

★ **Share what you have created with those around you** and be joyful in it! We are VERY proud of you!

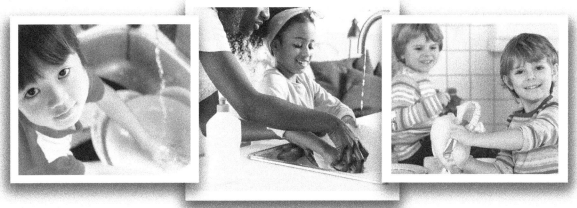

KITCHEN SAFETY AT HOME FOR KIDS

FACT: Cooking is serious business (and a TON of fun)!

<u>**FOR KIDS**</u>:

You'll be extra confident and have more fun when you understand kitchen hygiene and safety. Once you master these tips, your parents will feel more comfortable to stand back and watch you soar and explore in your kitchen!

Sticky Fingers Cooking's ABC Guide to Kitchen Safety:

(A) **Always** *Ask an Adult!*

(B) **Beware** *of Burners + Blades*

(C) **Clean** *your Clappers*

(D) **Do** *it as a Team*

(E) **Eat & Enjoy** *Everything (don't yuck my yum!)*

(F) <u>***FUN***</u> *is #1!*

Clean your clappers! Hygiene FIRST!

1. **Tie back your hair.** Make sure you don't have any loose clothing or dangling jewelry.

2. **Wear shoes!** Bare feet risk getting burned with hot mixtures or cut with sharp utensils.

3. **Wash your hands often!** Wash your hands for 20 seconds with soap and water.

Washing should be all the way up past your wrists and down to the tips of your fingertips. Sing "Happy Birthday" twice or the "ABC Song" once.

4. **Use a paper towel or clean cloth towel** to dry off and use that same towel to turn off the water faucet (the germs you shared with the faucet when you turned it on won't jump back on your hands this way!).

Techniques to keep your kitchen safe!

1. **Keep all electrical appliances away from water to avoid shocks!** Stay away from electrical sockets, especially if your hands are wet.

2. **Always begin by reading the complete recipe: be sure you understand the instructions.** Gather all your ingredients, utensils, and pans that you need before you start.

3. **Be very careful with knives**. Kitchen knives should be sharp. Sharp knives work the best and are safer because they cut through foods easily. Use the "bear claw," "bridge," and "plank"

methods for cutting food. Practice with an adult before you start cooking. Hold and carry all knives with the point side down and away from you. Don't put knives into soapy water in your sink because someone could reach in and get cut. In the dishwasher, place knives point side down.

4. **Don't put cooked food on an unwashed plate or cutting board that held raw food.** Always use a clean plate. Never taste uncooked food. Remember that raw eggs and flour can contain pathogenic bacteria, so don't taste any food with uncooked flour or eggs in it.

5. **Be careful when tasting hot food.** Foods from the oven should cool for at least 10 minutes for entrées and side dishes, 30 minutes for bread, and 20 minutes for cookies. If the recipe says to cool completely before serving… do it!

6. **Hot mixtures can burn really quickly.** Make sure that pot handles are turned away from the front of the stovetop. If the handles are hanging over the front of the stove, the pot with its hot contents could be knocked onto the floor, and on to you. Ouch.

7. **Use hot pads when removing food from the oven or microwave,** and never put hot food in your mouth or touch hot food.

8. **If you hurt yourself, tell an adult immediately.**

9. **Have a well-stocked first aid kit and a fire extinguisher** in the kitchen at all times.

10. **Keep paper towels, dish towels, and pot holders away from the range top so they don't catch on fire.** If a fire starts, call an adult immediately. NEVER put water on a kitchen fire. If the fire is small, throw baking soda on it to smother the flames. If the fire is in a pan, ask an adult to put the lid on the pan to remove oxygen from the fire to put it out. Use a fire extinguisher. If flames are large, call 911 and leave the house immediately.

Let's get COOKING!

1. **Always begin by reading the complete recipe**. Be sure you understand the instructions.

2. **Gather all your ingredients, utensils, and pans** that you need before you start.

Wrap it up! A clean kitchen is a happy kitchen!

1. **When you're done cooking, clean the kitchen.** No complaints! This means wipe up spills, place utensils and bowls in the dishwasher, clean pans, and put away all of your ingredients.

2. **Not only is keeping your kitchen clean important for safety and hygiene**, but your parents will be proud of your acting so grown up and so responsible that you will be invited to cook up even more fun in your kitchen!

"Wow, this is really crazy good stuff I just made..!"
Jason, age 7

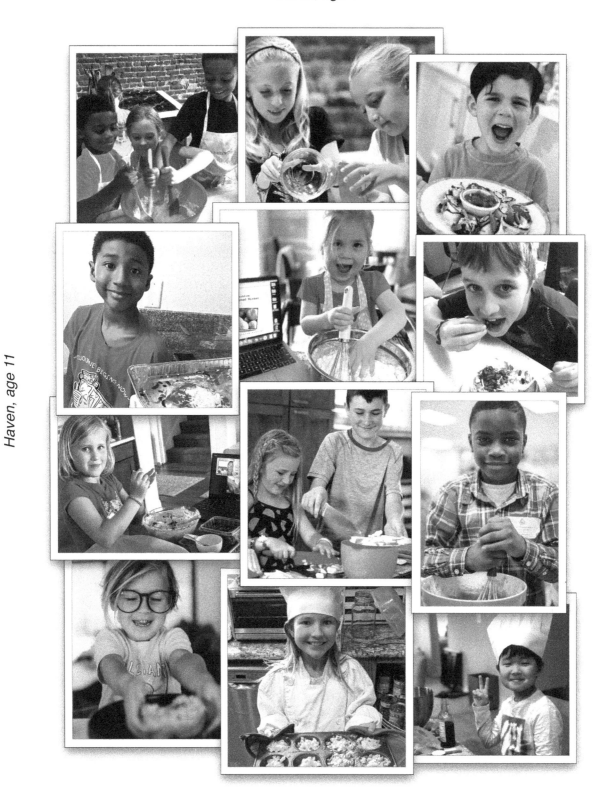

"This is so awesome; I love it!"
Haven, age 11

"I give this a hundred thumbs up!"
Phoebe, age 7

"My parents aren't going to believe I made this! It's so good! I LOVE COOKING!!"
Grayson, age 8

Shanghai Stir-Fried Chunky Noodles
+ Sautéed Bok Choy
+ Green Tea Shakes

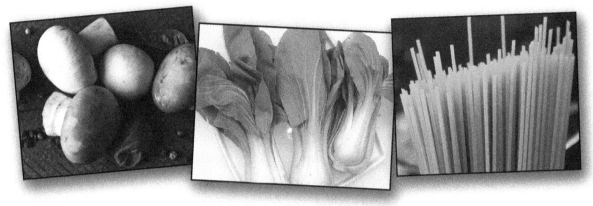

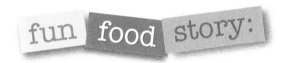

fun **food** story:

Knock! Knock!! Who's There? Bok. Bok Who? Didn't you hear me Bokking? I'm Bok Choy! Eating long noodles with your friends and family to celebrate the new year is considered good luck and will ensure happiness. Since the Chinese words for "face" (*miàn*) and "noodle" (*mein*) sound the same, it eventually came to be that people ate long noodles to symbolize a long face and, therefore, long life.

This recipe is everything that I LOVE about preparing and eating food with kids. It brings together food, fun, family, tradition, and history wrapped up into a beautiful and healthy bowl of steaming noodles. My kids love to order Shanghai Noodles when we eat out at Chinese restaurants. Our kids immediately devour those noodles, ignoring everything else on the table.

These Shanghai Stir-Fried Noodles are super easy to prepare, with only a few ingredients, and very addictive! It'll be done and on the table within 15-20 minutes—and everyone in your family will love it. If you're not a vegetarian/vegan, simply add your favorite meats into the dish. *Měiwèi*—"yummy" in Mandarin Chinese!

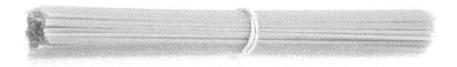

shanghai stir-fried chunky noodles

ingredients

1 lb Asian wheat noodles (like Lo Mein or Udon

1 C firm tofu, mushrooms, or 2 eggs

3 T soy sauce (or tamari)

2 tsp rice wine or red wine vinegar

1/2 tsp cornstarch

1/2 to 3/4 lb (2 to 3 C) bok choy

2 stalks green onions

clove garlic

1 to 2 carrots

2 T vegetable oil

1/2 to 1 tsp sugar/honey/agave nectar

pinch of black pepper

cook+cut+crack

Cook **1 lb Asian wheat noodles (like Lo Mein or Udon)** according to package directions. Drain and toss in a bit of oil to prevent sticking! Meanwhile, have your kids prep your choice of **1 cup firm tofu, 1 cup mushrooms,** or **2 eggs.** Cut either the tofu or mushrooms as evenly as possible into slices. If using eggs, crack eggs into a small bowl and whisk.

measure+mix+marinate

In a medium bowl, combine ½ **T soy sauce, 2 tsp rice wine or red wine vinegar,** and ½ **tsp cornstarch** and mix well. Add the chopped tofu or mushrooms, if using, and marinate until ready to stir fry. If using eggs, pour the marinade into the eggs and whisk well.

chop+grate

Have your kids chop up ½ **to ¾ lb (2 to 3 C) bok choy, 2 stalks green onions,** and **1 clove garlic.** Grate **1-2 carrots.** Combine the onion, garlic, and carrot in one bowl and keep the bok choy separate.

measure+combine

In a small bowl, have your kids measure and combine **2½ T soy sauce, 2 T vegetable oil, ½ to 1 tsp sugar/honey/agave nectar**, and **a pinch of black pepper**. Set aside.

heat+sauté

Heat **1 T oil** in a nonstick skillet or wok over medium-high heat on your stovetop. Once the oil is warmed, add the prepared tofu, mushrooms, or egg with its marinade, as well as the prepared carrots, garlic, and green onions, and sauté. When the tofu, vegetables, and/or eggs are just cooked, remove from the skillet and set aside. Next, add your cooked noodles and the soy sauce mixture into the hot skillet and sauté/stir-fry until piping hot.

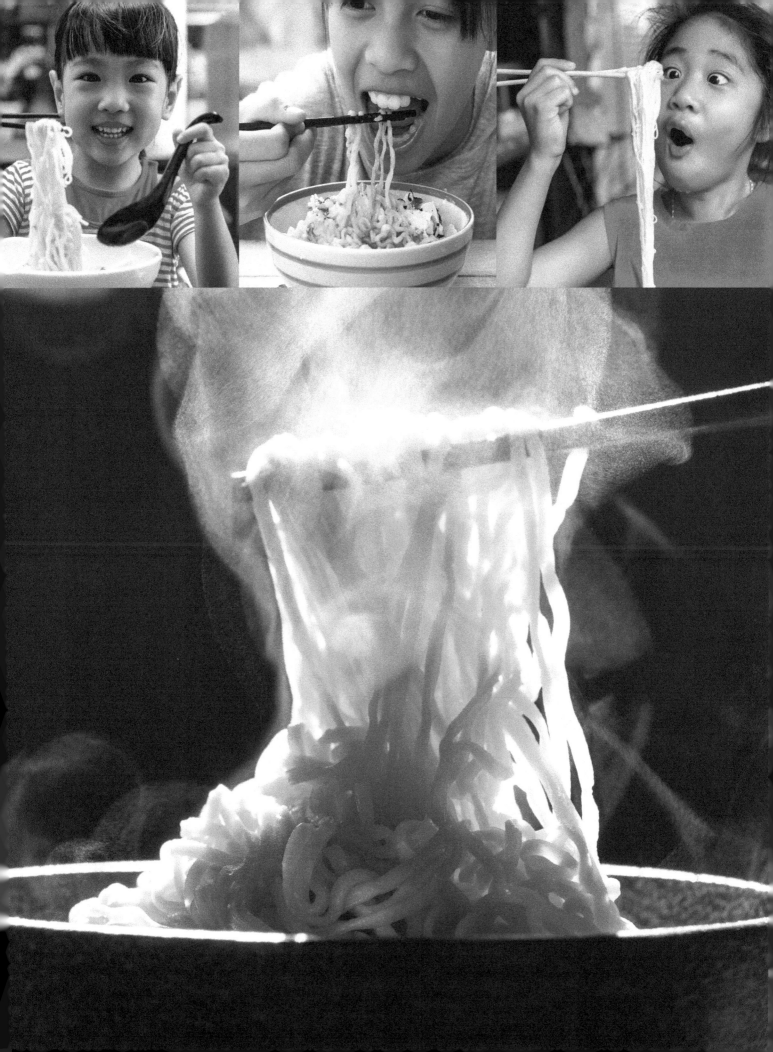

green tea honey shakes

ingredients

1 to 2 bags decaf green tea

3 T honey/sugar/agave nectar

2 C vanilla yogurt

4 C ice

steep+discard+dissolve

Heat **1 cup water** and pour into a pitcher or large heatproof cup with **1-2 decaf green tea** bags. Steep for 5 minutes, remove and discard the tea bags. Have your kids stir **3 T honey/sugar/ agave** into the tea until completely dissolved. Set to the side to cool.

add+blend

Add **2 cup vanilla yogurt** and **4 cup ice**. Blend with your blender or an immersion blender in a pitcher until smooth, thick, and creamy.

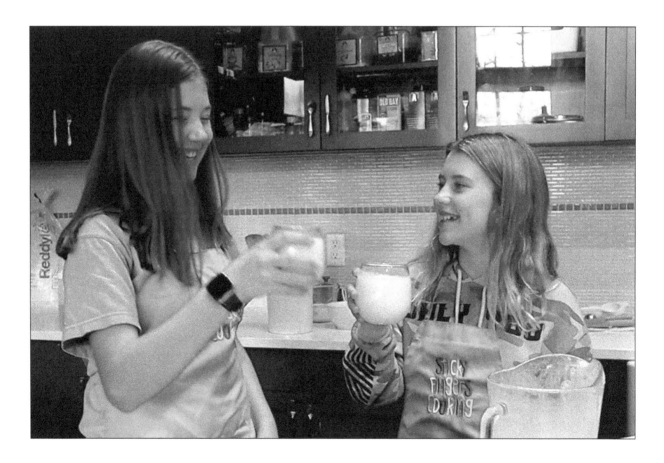

ASIA — Shanghai Stir-Fried Chunky Noodles

Singapore
Curry Street Noodles
+ Singapore
Zinger-Slingers

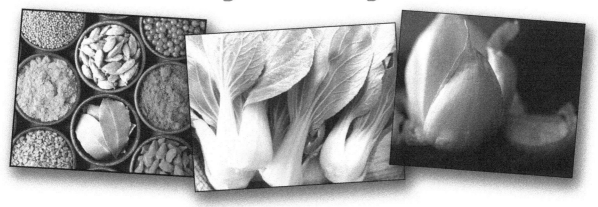

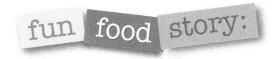

The Curious History of Curry

Curry derives from the language of the Tamil people in South Asia; the word *kari* originally referred to sauce but was later changed to *curry*. Curry powder is a actually blend of spices rather than a single spice, and the spice level of the blend can be adjusted. It is used in the cuisine of almost every country and can be incorporated into a dish or even a drink.

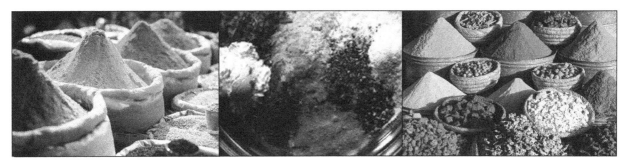

Curry is one of the oldest spice mixes and is most often associated with Indian cuisine. Most recipes and producers of curry powder usually include coriander, turmeric, cumin, fenugreek, and red pepper in their blends. Depending on the recipe, additional ingredients such as ginger, garlic, asafoetida, fennel seed, caraway, cinnamon, clove, mustard seed, green cardamom, black cardamom, nutmeg, long pepper, and black pepper may also be added. It should be remembered that curry powder is more of a generic term for a blend of different spices.

The Featured Ingredient: Bok Choy

★ **Bok choy is classified as a cabbage**, sometimes even called Chinese cabbage. Bok choy is a distant relative of broccoli, cabbage, and cauliflower. However, bok choy bears little resemblance to the round cabbages found in most supermarkets. It has glossy, dark-green leaves and thick, crisp white stalks in a loose head. Its white stalks resemble celery without the stringiness, while the leaves of the most common variety are similar to romaine lettuce or spinach.

★ **Bok choy is a fast growing vegetable.** It is ready to harvest in only 6 to 7 weeks after sowing.

★ **Bok choy's popularity comes from its light, sweet flavor**, crisp texture, and nutritional value. The yellow flowering center (head) is especially prized.

★ **Bok choy is found in soups, stir-fries, appetizers, salads, sides, and main dishes.** The smaller varieties are valued for their tenderness. Bok choy is one of those good-for-you vegetables that can be eaten raw, quick-cooked, steamed, stir-fried, or boiled.

★ **Bok choy is nutritious and high in vitamin A, vitamin C, potassium, and calcium.** Their leaves are higher in vitamin content and flavor than stalks which have a mild taste, similar to Swiss chard or romaine lettuce. Bok choy has all the benefits of a leafy green: calcium, magnesium, vitamin A, vitamin C, and Folate.

The Tasty and Diverse Street Foods of Singapore

Singapore's diverse street food cuisine is a delicious reason to visit this culturally unique city state. Fresh local fruits and vegetables are prepared in an array of delicious dishes generally related to a particular ethnic group—Chinese, Malay, and Indian.

Though many cultures have an extensive variety of delectable street foods, the food stalls of Hawker Centre in Singapore are truly unique. In 2018, there were 114 hawker centers maintained by the National Environment Agency; two of these stalls were the first in the world to receive the coveted Michelin Star award.

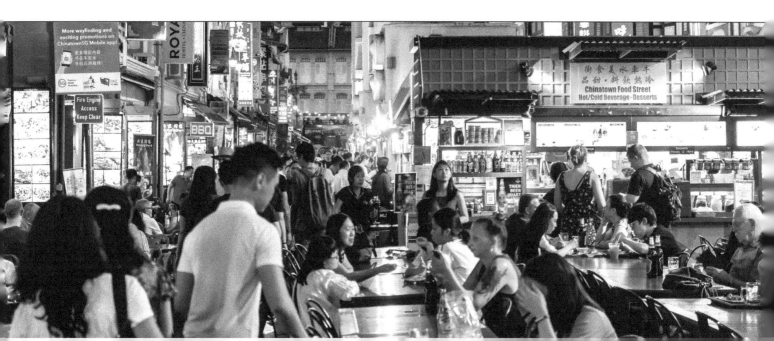

Singapore curry street noodles

ingredients

8 oz dried Asian rice vermicelli (thin) noodles

1 to 2 bunches baby bok choy

2 medium cloves garlic

4 medium green onions stalks

½ C bean sprouts

4 T low-sodium soy sauce

4 T low-sodium soy sauce

2 T rice vinegar

1 T + 1 tsp brown sugar or honey

2 eggs

6 T vegetable oil

2 T mild curry powder

1 tsp turmeric

pre-soak+drain

Soak **8 ounces dried Asian rice vermicelli noodles** in hot water for 15 minutes, or until softened. Drain the water and set aside.

chop+snap

Have your children chop up **1-2 baby bok choy**, **2 medium cloves garlic**, **4 medium green onions** and **½ C bean sprouts** in half. If you choose any optional vegetables from the shopping list, have your kids cut and or grate them now. Set everything to the side.

measure+whisk

Measure and whisk **4 T low-sodium soy sauce**, **2 T rice vinegar**, and **1 T + 1 tsp brown sugar or honey** in a bowl together. Add the pre-chopped green onions into the soy sauce bowl. Set aside.

crack+beat

Crack open **2 eggs** into a bowl and season with salt and black pepper. Lightly beat the eggs.

heat+cook

Heat your non-stick skillet over medium high heat. Carefully pour in 1 **T of oil**. Add the beaten eggs and cook just like scrambled eggs. Take the eggs out of the skillet when they are fully cooked and set to the side.

stir-fry+sprinkle

Add **4 T of oil** and add the pre-chopped garlic and bok choy. Stir-fry the vegetables for 2 to 3 minutes, or until the vegetables are softened. Add **bean sprouts (and any other vegetables you are using)** and sprinkle in **2 T mild curry powder** and **1 tsp turmeric** and cook 1 to 2 minutes more.

pour+toss+taste

Turn the heat to low. Gently pour in the soy sauce mixture into the skillet, and toss with vegetables. Then add the softened (pre-soaked) **Asian rice vermicelli noodles** and the egg (if using), and toss to combine. Stir-fry 2 to 3 minutes, or until noodles absorb some of the sauce and soften. Remove from heat. Taste. Does it need more salt? More sugar? More soy sauce? More curry? Then eat and shout *Sangat lazat*, which means "it is very delicious" in Malay!

zinger-slingers

ingredients

1 C pineapple

handful fresh cherries (optional)

12-oz can ginger ale (or Stevia soda)

2 C ice

sugar or honey (only if needed)

chop+pit

Have your kids chop up **1 C pineapple**, either fresh or canned, and add to your blender. Show your kids how to take out the pits from a **small handful of fresh cherries** and add to your blender.

open+pour+enjoy

Open and pour in **12 oz can ginger ale** (we use Stevia soda) and about **2 cups ice cubes** into your blender. Blend until smooth. Taste the Singapore Zinger-Slinger (adjust with Stevia, honey or sugar if needed) and enjoy with your noodles!

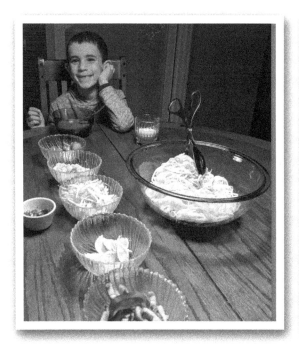
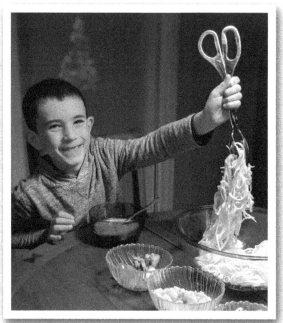

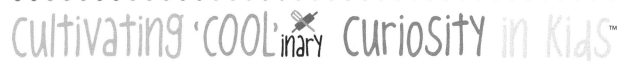

thyme for a fun activity

Spectacular Spice Paint

Ingredients:

Ground aromatic spices of
your choice such as turmeric,
cinnamon, ginger, nutmeg,
smoked paprika, etc.

Supplies:

Paintbrush(es)
Paper
Paint tray(s)
Water

Smell and memory are closely linked; often just a whiff of certain smells can trigger memories from long ago. This easy activity offers the opportunity to make memories, so that maybe one day years from now, you might catch a whiff of turmeric or cinnamon and think back to those days of painting with spices

Directions

- **Start by prepping your paint space.** Painting outdoors can be a unique experience for kids, and you don't have to worry too much about any potential mess! If you are painting indoors, it might be helpful to lay down newspapers, tape down a large plastic bag to the table, or set up to paint in a baking tray for easy cleanup!

- **Have fun gently smelling and selecting your favorite spices!** If you want to use whole spices such as mustard seed or fenugreek seed, try grinding them into a powder with a coffee grinder.

- **Add a small amount of each spice** into separate paint trays, bowls, paper cups, or a recycled egg carton.

- **Then, slowly mix a small amount of water into each spice until you get a paint-like consistency.** The less water you add, the more vibrant in color your paint will be. While painting, be sure to smell the aromatic art you're creating and memories you're making!

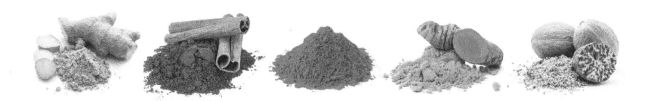

India's Turnip Tikka Masala
+ Street-Style Hakka Noodles
+ Classic Indian Sweet
Yogurt Lassi

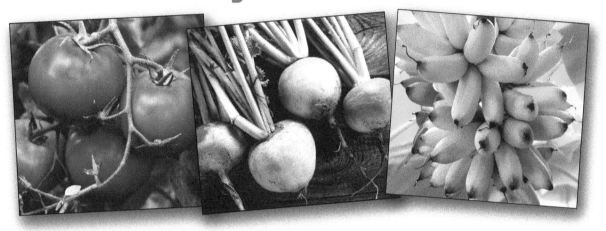

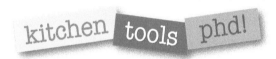

Slicing, Chopping, Mincing, Blending!

SLICE: To cut into pieces using a sawing motion with your knife!

CHOP: To cut food into rough pieces that are not usually the same size!

MINCE: To cut food into tiny pieces!

BLEND: The action of mixing or combining things together.

What Can We Learn About Turnips?

Turnips may LOOK like potatoes, but they're actually not related to potatoes at all! Turnips are related to radishes, mustard greens, broccoli, cauliflower, and collard greens! They're a member of the Brassicaceae Family. Smell them—they smell spicy like radishes! They have a sweet, peppery, slightly spicy flavor.

★ **Before people carved pumpkins into jack-o-lanterns** on Halloween, they carved turnips!

★ **The origin of turnips is uncertain,** though it's believed to be somewhere in Asia or Europe.

★ **Turnips are rich in vitamin C and potassium!** The leafy part of the plant contains more nutrients compared to the root. Both vitamin C and potassium are essential for heart health!

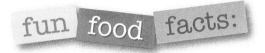

What the heck are Tikka Masala and Hakka Noodles?

Tikka masala is a dish made of marinated chunks of chicken in a creamy red-orange sauce. Though its origin isn't certain, the most popular view is that the dish was invented by an Indian migrant chef, most likely somewhere in the United Kingdom. While not considered a traditional Indian dish, tikka masala has become one of the most popular dishes throughout the United Kingdom. It was invented, they say, to satisfy the British people's preference to have meat cooked and served in some kind of gravy.

Hakka noodles originated when Chinese people settled in Kolkata and developed a new cuisine by adding Indian spices to their traditional foods, like noodles. Hakka noodles became world famous. They're loved for their flavor combination of Indian spices and Chinese sauces.

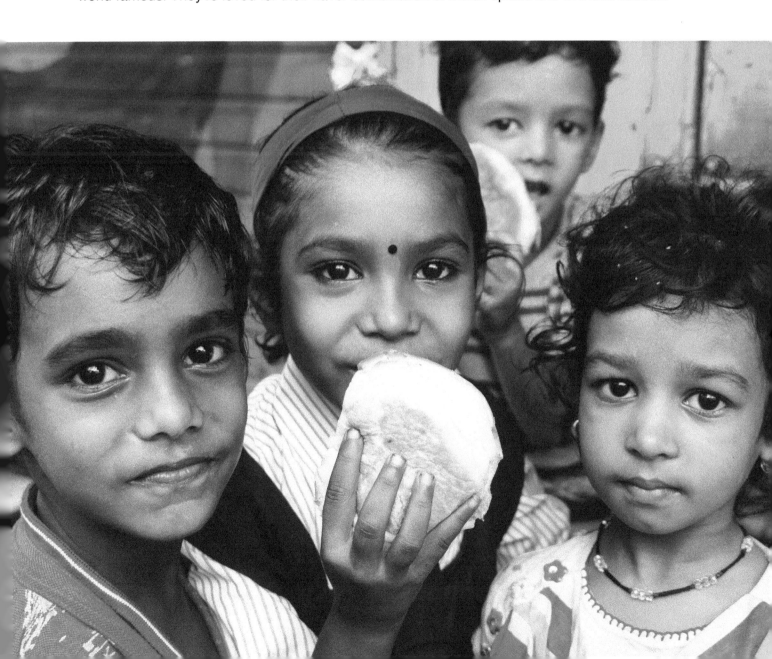

india's turnip tikka masala

ingredients

1 green onion
1 clove garlic
1 carrot
2 small turnips
1 Yukon gold or red potato
1 14 oz can diced tomatoes
1 -2 T garam masala seasoning

1½ T garam masala
1 14-oz can chopped tomatoes
2 tsp sugar
1½ tsp salt
1 ripe banana

snip+grate+mince+chop

Use a pair of clean scissors to snip **1 green onion** into small bits. Peel and grate 1 large carrot carefully using a box grater. Peel and mince **1 clove garlic.** Chop **2 small turnips** and 1 Yukon gold potato into 1-inch pieces.

melt+sauté+add+stir

Melt **2 T butter** in a large skillet. Sauté the onion, garlic, and carrot. Stir in **1 ½ T garam masala** spice mixture. Add chopped turnips and potato and stir to coat in the spice mixture.

Then add ½ **C water, 1 14-oz can chopped tomatoes, 2 tsp sugar, 1 ½ tsp salt.** Stir and cover the skillet. Turn heat to low and let simmer. Meanwhile, boil **8 oz angel hair pasta** for the Street-Style Hakka Noodles!

chop+add+stir

Chop **1 banana** into very small bits. Add to the skillet and cook for 1 more minute, uncovered. Taste and add more seasoning as necessary. Serve over fried Street-Style Hakka Noodles and ENJOY!

street-style hakka noodles

ingredients

8 oz angel hair pasta
1 T olive oil, and more for drizzling
1 clove garlic
1-inch piece of peeled, fresh ginger

3 green onions
2 T soy sauce
1 tsp sugar
1 T vinegar

boil+snap+drizzle

Boil **6 C water** in a sauce pot. Snap **8 oz angel hair pasta** in half and add to the boiling water. Boil for 3 minutes, then drain and drizzle noodles with **olive oil** to keep them from sticking.

mince+grate+snip

Mince **1 clove garlic**, grate **1-inch piece of peeled fresh ginger**, and snip **3 green onions** into thin pieces.

measure+whisk+sauté

Measure and whisk together **2 T soy sauce**, **1 tsp sugar**, and **1 T vinegar**. Add **1 T olive oil** to a medium-sized skillet and sauté the garlic, ginger, and onions for 30 seconds. Add the boiled angel hair pasta and soy sauce mixture to the skillet. Break up the noodles with a spatula to coat them in the sauce. Serve noodles topped with your tasty Turnip Tikka Masala and ENJOY!

classic indian sweet yogurt lassi

ingredients

2 ripe bananas

2 T sugar

½ C cream or yogurt

2 C ice

chop+measure+blend+pour

Peel and chop **2 ripe bananas** and add to a blender. Measure and add **2 T sugar**, **½ C cream or yogurt** and **2 C ice**. Blend until the mixture is thick and smooth, adding more cream, yogurt, or water if you need to thin it out some. Pour into cups and CHEERS!

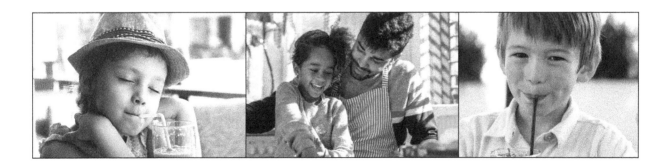

Very Vietnamese Veggie Bánh Mì Sandwiches + Hibiscus Ginger Party Punch

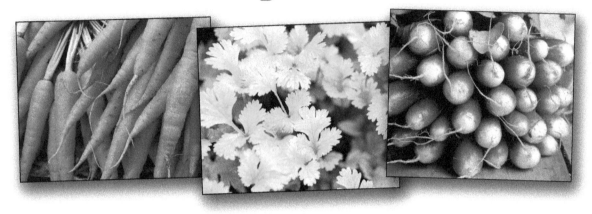

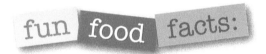

The Fascinating History of Bánh Mì

The Bánh Mì (baan mee) sandwich is a wonderful example of the fusion of two great cultures, the Vietnamese and the French. During colonial times, the French gained power over Vietnam, and though many people believe there was no benefit to French oversight, they can agree the legacy of the *Bánh Mì* sandwich is a happy one. The original sandwich crafted in Saigon consisted of just butter and ham or pate on a bageutte.

The word *bánh* generally refers to food made with flour, and the sandwich was known to locals as *Báhn Tay*. Expensive delis sold the sandwich to the wealthy, making the dish too expensive for the working-class to afford. In the mid-20th century, the sandwich became known as *Báhn Mì*, and local Vietnamese started to make it truly their own after French control ceased. Egg-based mayonnaise replaced butter, and local flavors and ingredients like pickled vegetables made this dish shine.

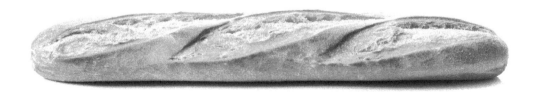

The featured ingredient: Radishes!

★ **The word *radish* is derived from the Latin word for "root."**

★ **Radishes belong to the Brassicaceae family and the genus Raphanus.** Raphanus comes from the Greek *raphanos*, meaning "quickly appearing," which makes sense since this vegetable is known for growing rapidly in the garden!

★ **Radishes are known for their naturally-cooling characteristic and strong flavor.** Eastern medicine practices utilize radishes to lower excess body heat during the warmer months.

★ **They are a hydrating vegetable due to their high water content.** The phosphorus and zinc present, coupled with the water content, make radishes nourishing for the body's tissues and skin.

★ **Because of their pungent flavor, radishes can help clear the sinuses and relieve common cold symptoms.** Their high vitamin C content can also help fight off viruses!

★ **Radishes can have a calming effect on the digestive system.** They break down and remove toxins and free radicals from the body.

★ **As a cruciferous vegetable, radishes are relatives of broccoli and cabbage.** They are also related to wasabi, a type of horseradish, which isn't too surprising considering the spicy flavor of both vegetables.

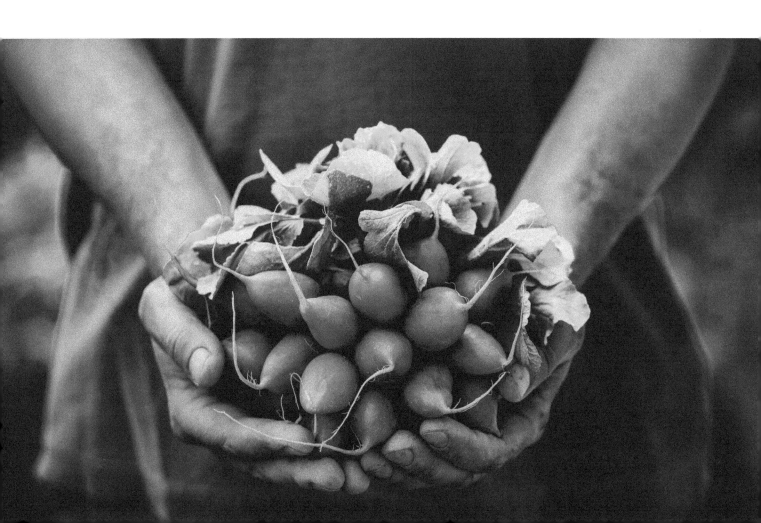

very vietnamese veggie báhn mi sandwiches

ingredients

2 fresh French baguettes
(for GF, use GF bread, lettuce wraps, or rice paper)
mayonnaise
2 carrots
4-6 radishes (or 2-4 inches Daikon radish)
½ small cucumber
½ block tofu (or 2 eggs)
2 T oil

small handful cilantro
soy sauce
lime (optional)
½ C water
¼ C sugar or honey
¼ C white or rice vinegar
½ T salt
1 clove garlic
½ inch fresh ginger

peel+measure+combine

First, we'll make the pickles, starting with the marinade. Have your kids carefully peel ½ **inch fresh ginger** and **1 clove garlic**. In a cold skillet or saucepan on the stovetop, combine ½ **C water**, ¼ **C sugar or honey**, ¼ **C white vinegar or rice vinegar**, ½ **T salt**, and the whole peeled ginger and garlic.

heat+dissolve

Heat the marinade to almost a boil and stir until the sugar or honey has dissolved, about 1 minute. Allow the mixture to cool.

grate+squeeze

Have your kids carefully grate **2 carrots**, ½ **of a cucumber**, and **4-6 radishes**. Place the vegetables in a clean towel (or paper towels) and squeeze out the extra liquid. Place grated vegetables in a bowl.

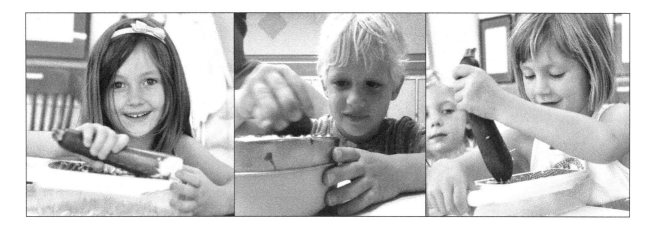

pour+marinate

Pour the cooled marinade over the grated vegetables and set aside to marinate for 10-40 minutes.

crumble+sauté

Heat some oil in a nonstick skillet on your stovetop and have your kids crumble ½ **block of tofu**. Sauté the tofu until it is a little brown over medium/high heat. Season with some dashes of **soy sauce** to taste and remove from heat. (Alternatively, scramble 2 eggs.)

slice+pull+assemble

Slice **2 baguettes** in half, the long way, and have your kids pull some of the center of the bread out of the baguette halves, leaving a little cavity for the filling. Drain and rinse (or squeeze) off the marinade from the vegetable pickles. To assemble the Bánh Mì, have your kids spread each half of the **2 baguettes** with some mayonnaise and fill the cavity of the bottom half of the bread with the tofu (or egg), the pickled vegetables, some torn **cilantro leaves**, and a **squeeze of lime juice**. Top with the other half of the baguette. Cut the sandwiches into equal parts and EAT!

● ●

hibiscus ginger party punch

ingredients

4 C water
1-2 inches fresh ginger
1 to 2 bags hibiscus tea bags

½ C sugar or honey (or 2 packs of Stevia)
lime (optional)

boil+peel+combine

Boil **4 C of water**. Meanwhile, have your kids carefully peel **1-2 inches of fresh ginger** and set to the side. Measure and combine **1-2 hibiscus tea bags, ½ C sugar or honey (or 2 packs of stevia)** and the fresh peeled ginger in a pitcher. Slowly pour the boiling hot water into the drink pitcher.

infuse+strain

Set your pitcher aside for 15-30 minutes to let the mixture infuse. Strain out the tea bags and ginger before serving. Serve in cups poured over ice and enjoy!

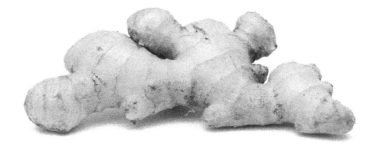

Let's Learn Some Vietnamese While We Cook!

1... **một (mohk)** – like a Buddhist monk

2... **hai (high)** – Like as high as airplanes fly

3... **ba (bah)** – Like what a sheep says

4... **bốn (bone)** – Like what a dog chews on

5... **năm (nuhm)** – Like when your hands are cold and numb

6... **sáu (sao)** – Like when you sew

7... **bảy (bye)** – Like goodbye!

8... **tám (tahm)** – Like a TAMbourine

9... **chín (cheen)** – Like your chin

10... **mười (meui)** – Like what a cat says

Let's Finish with a Laugh!

What is the coolest vegetable in the garden?

A RADish!

Why are radishes so smart?

Because they're well-red!

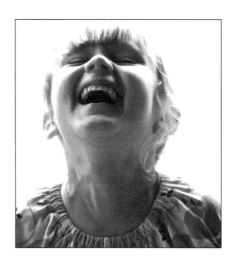

Outrageous Orange Cardamom Chai Cupcakes
+ Chai Glaze
+ Orange Chai Cream Soda

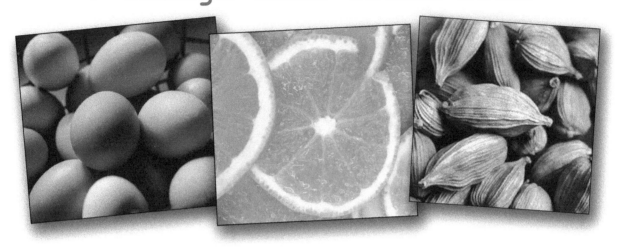

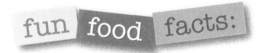

I am passionate about Indian chai spices. The combination of rich, aromatic spices can warm me up and calm me down at the same time. My daughters have developed a deep love for baking and trying new, creative flavors, so I thought we would combine chai (tea) and cupcakes together for this Sticky Fingers Cooking recipe!

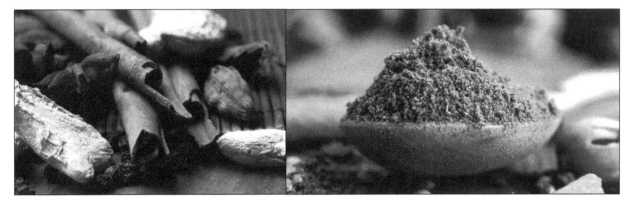

Did you know that after chocolate and vanilla, orange is the world's most popular flavor? Oranges have loads of nutrition yet are low in calories and contain no cholesterol or saturated fats. In addition to being a great source of vitamin C, oranges are also high in dietary fiber, vitamin A, potassium, and calcium, to name a few of their virtues.

For this recipe, I used the base of an orange cupcake recipe but infused the batter with chai spices. The sweet aroma of the baked cupcakes made me immediately fall head over heels for this recipe, and my daughters could not agree more. We double dipped them in a sweet, spicy chai glaze for good measure and added a fun, healthy twist with a homemade, orange cream soda to round it all out. Whether you're craving something sweet or a Chai Tea Latte, I'm pretty sure I've got you covered! SAY: *Svādiṣṭa!* That means "delicious" in Hindi.

Have fun + happy, healthy cooking! - Chef Erin

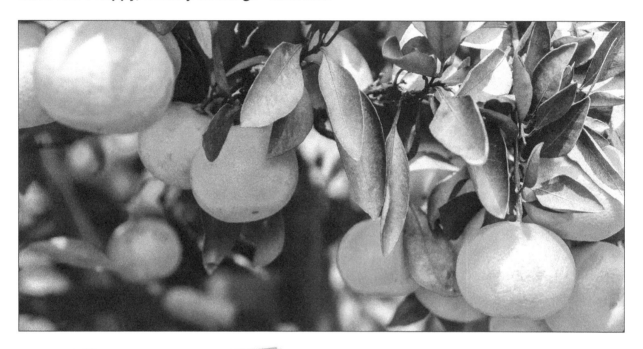

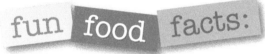

What Is Chai?

Although it is common in the US to use the word "chai tea," *chai* **(derived from** *chá* **in Mandarin Chinese) is actually the word for tea in many languages.** Chai has been enjoyed as a beverage for thousands of years and dates back to ancient India and Siam. Besides water, it is the most popular drink in the world.

Chai is made of finely ground tea leaves and a blend of spices and herbs. Depending on where you travel, each chai blend might look a little different, and families tend to have their own secret recipe for making chai. Generally, though, chai includes warm spices like ginger, cinnamon, cardamom, cloves, and star anise.

Eastern and Ayurvedic medicine use chai for its natural healing qualities. Ginger is known for its anti-inflammatory properties while cinnamon can help lower blood pressure and blood sugar. Chai is good for the immune system, digestive system, and the heart!

It is believed that Chai comes from the leaves of tea plants in Western China, Tibet, and Northern India. According to legend, the Chinese emperor Shen Nung accidentally discovered chai leaves thousands of years ago. One day, he journeyed into the mountains to study plants and herbs for their medicinal qualities. While he was sitting under a tree in a forest boiling water, a few leaves fell from overhead and landed in the water. The emperor later tasted the concoction and fell in love with it. Other versions of the story say he drank tea to detoxify his body after testing various medicinal herbs on himself.

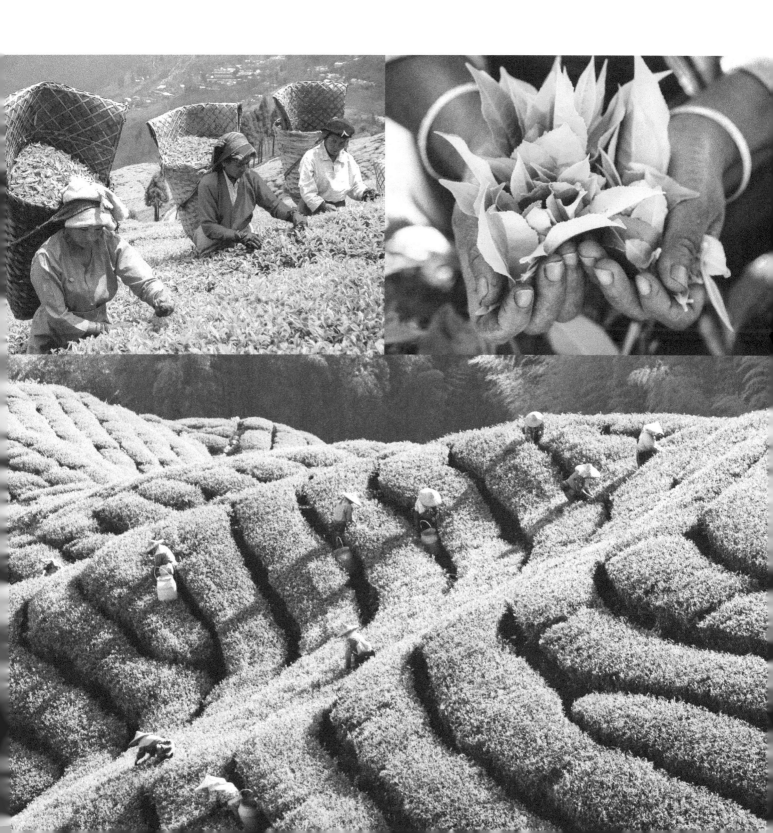

outrageous orange cardamom chai cupcakes

ingredients

1 bag decaf chai tea

2 C all-purpose flour

1½ tsp baking powder

½ tsp salt

½ tsp ground cardamom

½ C butter, room temperature

1¼ C granulated white sugar

2 large eggs

1 tsp pure vanilla extract

¼ C milk

1 orange

pre-brew+pre-heat+pre-line

Prepare 1 C of tea from **decaf Chai tea bag** with boiling water, set to the side to steep for up to 15 minutes and let cool to room temperature. The longer you steep the tea, the stronger the flavor. Pre-heat your oven to 350 degrees and have kids line your muffin tin with paper liners.

whisk+beat

In a medium bowl, have kids whisk together **2 C all purpose flour, 1½ tsp baking powder, ½ tsp salt** and **½ tsp ground cardamom.** In a large bowl, cream together ½ **C room temperature butter** and 1¼ **C sugar** until fluffy and light. Beat in **2 large eggs**, one at a time, followed by **2 tsp vanilla extract**. Add in ¼ **C milk**, followed by the cup of pre-made tea. (Reserve 3 to 4 T for chai tea glaze and orange chai cream soda.)

zest+juice

Zest the peel from **1 orange** and fold into the batter and then squeeze the juice into the batter. Mix only until all ingredients are combined and no streaks of flour remain. Then fill the pre-lined muffin tin with the batter about ¾ full.

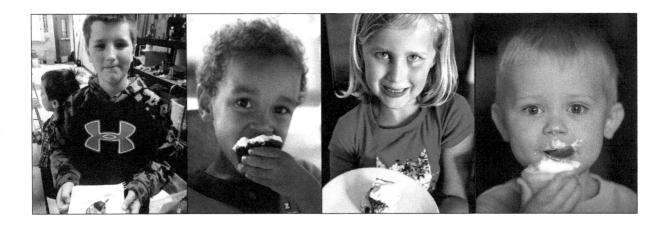

bake+cool

Bake in pre-heated oven for 15-20 minutes at 350 F, or until a toothpick inserted into the center comes out clean. Let your cupcakes cool completely before adding the glaze.

● ●

chai tea glaze

ingredients

1 C powdered sugar

1-2 T reserved chai tea, pre-brewed

1 Ziploc-type bag

measure+smoosh+glaze

Have kids measure the 1 **C powdered sugar** and the **pre-brewed Chai tea** into a **Ziploc-type bag** and SMOOSH all around until a glaze forms. Snip the corner of the bag to glaze the cupcakes!

● ●

orange chai cream soda

ingredients

1 orange

12 packs of Stevia (or ¼ C sugar)

ice

1 liter sparkling mineral water

2 T reserved chai tea, brewed

1 tsp vanilla extract

measure+stir+enjoy

Cut the **orange** in half and squeeze the juice into a pitcher. Next, open up the **12 packs of stevia** (or use ¼ cup of sugar). Add **ice** and top with **1 liter sparkling mineral water**, **2 T of pre-brewed chai tea** and **1 tsp vanilla extract**.Stir and serve with the cupcakes!

thyme for a fun activity

Tea-Dyed Coffee Filter Art

Ingredients:
5 tea bags of each tea you chose
coffee filters

Supplies:
Large pot of water
Tray
Pencil

Tea has been used as a natural dye for fabrics for centuries. Bring some old-world charm to your home by using tea-dyed coffee filters to make a number of creative household decorations! You can practically use any kind of tea you have in your house: black, green, hibiscus, herbal. Generally, the stronger the tea smells, the stronger the color will be.

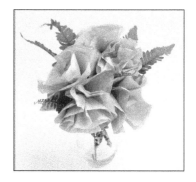

- **To start, bring to boil a large pot of water and then add 5 tea bags of your choice, letting the bags boil for about 10 minutes.** This will encourage the tea leaves to release a stronger color.

- **Then, turn off the stove and steep your coffee filters in the tea water for about 5-10 minutes.** The longer you let the filters steep, the deeper the color you'll achieve.

- **Carefully remove the filters from the pot and leave to dry;** you can either clip them to hang dry, or place them on a tray lined with paper towels. Before using the dyed coffee filters, ensure they have completely dried.

- **Try building a flower bouquet,** using the filters as the petals and pipe cleaners wound around a pencil for the stems, or use the filters to create a wreath or strand of garland—the possibilities are endless!

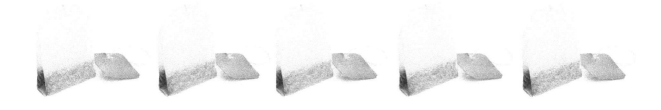

Mighty Mongolian Fried Rice
+ Cumin Frizzled Onions
+ Warm Mongolian Cinnamon
Milk Tea

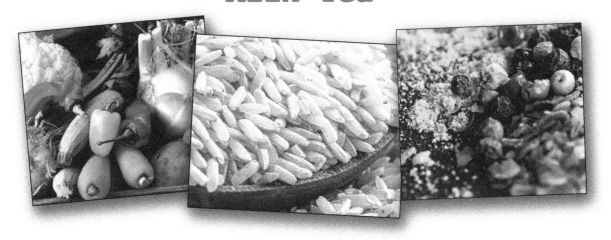

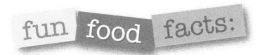

fun food facts:

★ **A spice is a seed, fruit, root, bark,** or other part of a plant mainly used to flavor, color or preserve a food.

★ **Spices are different from herbs.** Spices come from practically every part of a plant or tree except the leaf: root, stem, fruit, flower, seed, and/or bark. Herbs are the leafy parts of a plant.

★ **Not only do spices help food TASTE amazing, they also have amazing health benefits.**

★ **Turmeric helps the heart stay healthy** and protects our brains from losing memory.

★ **Black pepper helps with digestion** so that our bodies can utilize all the vitamins they need from the food we eat.

★ **Ginger is pungent and aromatic with citrus and earthy flavor notes.** It is often used to help calm upset stomachs.

★ **Cumin is earthy, nutty, spicy, and warm.** Cumin can help with digestion and calm upset stomachs. Cumin is good for the heart, too!

★ **The Spice Trade happened between the ancient civilizations of Asia, Northeast Africa, and Europe.** In ancient times, the region of Arabia supplied the Roman Empire with goods like cinnamon, cassia (similar to cinnamon but stronger in flavor), and other prized spices.

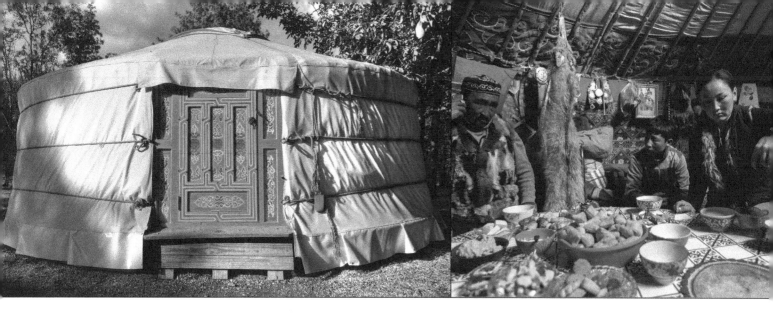

Let's Learn about Mongolia!

Genghis Khan is considered the founder of Mongolia which he ruled from 1206 until his death in 1227 CE. He unified forces and tribes throughout the Mongol Empire but used great force and violence to do so. Genghis Khan rose to power when he began unifying tribes scattered throughout northeast Asia, and he created the second largest empire of all time, bested only by the British Empire in the 1800s. Khan and his legion of horsemen conquered more in just 25 years than the Romans did in four hundred.

The Gobi Desert is the world's coldest desert and covers most of Southern Mongolia. The first dinosaur egg ever found was in the Gobi Desert!

Many Mongolians today live in yurts, or gers, which are tent-like, dome-shaped dwellings that are light enough to be disassembled, carried across the vast grasslands of Mongolia, and reassembled again.

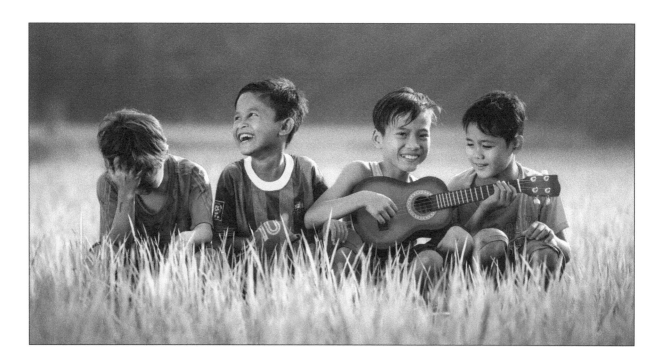

mighty mongolian fried rice

ingredients

1 C uncooked long-grain rice, rinsed and drained

½ tsp, and big pinch of salt

2 C mixed raw vegetables (broccoli, bell pepper, carrots, green beans, cauliflower, zucchini, mushrooms, or snap peas)

½ tsp each of ground cumin, coriander, paprika, turmeric, garlic or onion powder, and dried ginger

pinch of sugar

few shakes of black pepper

2 T butter or olive oil

measure+boil+cover+simmer

Measure **2 C water** and **1 C rinsed and drained long-grain rice** and add to a sauce pot. Add **½ tsp salt** and stir. Bring to a boil, then reduce heat to a simmer and cover. Rice takes about 15 mins to cook and is finished when all the water has evaporated and soaked into the rice. Turn off the heat and let sit covered for 10 minutes.

measure+mix+blend

While the rice cooks, dice **2 C of mixed vegetables**. Measure and add together: ½ **tsp cumin powder,** ½ **tsp turmeric,** ½ **tsp paprika,** ½ **tsp dried coriander,** ½ **tsp garlic or onion powder,** and ½ **tsp dried ginger**. Add a **big pinch of salt, a big pinch of sugar**, and a few shakes off **black pepper** to a small bowl. Mix to blend the spices.

chop+snap

To a large sauté pan, add **2 T butter or olive oil.** Add the diced veggies and sauté for a few minutes until crisp and tender. Sprinkle spices over the veggies and stir. Then add the cooked rice to the sauté pan and stir until the rice and veggies are combined. Top with the Cumin Frizzled Onions and enjoy!

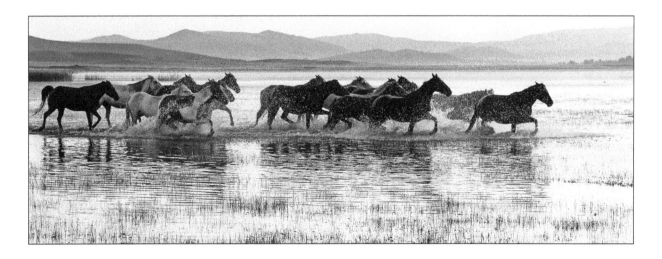

cumin frizzled onions

ingredients

4 green onions
1 T butter or olive oil

¼ tsp dried cumin
pinches of salt and sugar

snip+heat+sauté

Wash and snip **4 green onions** into thin slices using a clean set of scissors. Heat **1 T butter or olive oil** in a small skillet. Add the **green onions, ¼ tsp dried cumin**, and pinches of **salt and sugar** and sauté over medium heat until onions are slightly crispy and frizzled! Top Mighty Mongolian Fried Rice with Cumin Frizzled Onions and eat!

warm mongolian cinnamon milk tea

ingredients

2 C whole milk
2 C water
¼ C sugar or honey

pinches of cinnamon and salt
2 decaf tea bags (any flavor)

measure+add+boil

Measure and add **2 cups water, 2 cups whole milk, ¼ cup sugar or honey,** and **pinches of salt and ground cinnamon** to a sauce pot and bring to a soft boil.

simmer+steep+pour

Reduce heat to a simmer, then add **2 decaf tea bags** to the pot. Turn off the head and let the tea bags steep for 10 minutes. Pour into mugs and enjoy!

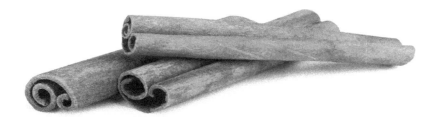

Let's Finish with a Laugh!

When do you put paprika in fried rice?

On Fry-days!

What do teapots wear to a tea party?

T-shirts!

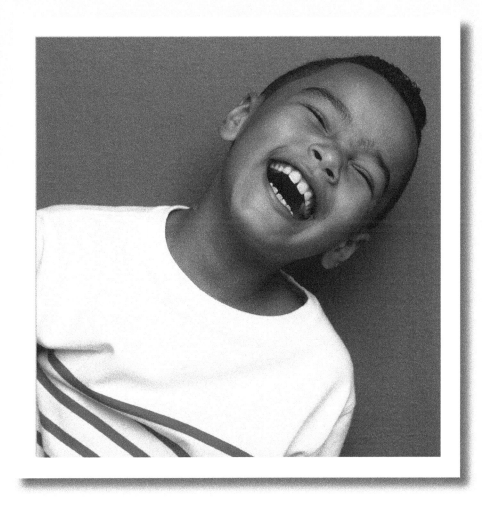

Terrific Temaki Sushi
手巻き寿司
+ Sweet Soy + Sparkling
Green Tea Soda

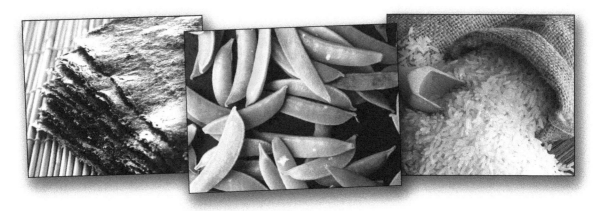

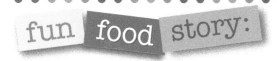

Hurry up and eat, kids. Your sushi is getting cold! If our family could eat sushi every day, we would. And we would be broke. While sushi is one of the healthiest foods you can eat, it is quite expensive when ordering from a restaurant.

Do you know what the word sushi really means? You may be surprised to know that the word sushi has nothing to do with raw fish; it means "it's sour." Literally. Sushi refers to the superstar ingredient found in all forms of sushi preparations: the sweetened vinegared rice!

The pearly white rolls, wraps, mounds, balls, and rounds of sweet-sour, barely warm, toothsome rice is the TRUE essence of sushi. Like other rice dishes across the world (paella, arroz con pollo, risotto, biryani, and the like), sushi is another creative way of taking a familiar and inexpensive food and adding a bit of something else interesting to make it new and truly unique.

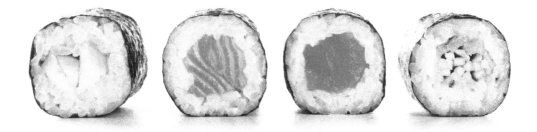

I've always believed that to be a great cook should not require tons of specialized kitchen equipment. You don't need to own a sushi rolling mat. You don't need to cut your rolls into perfectly measured rounds. Gosh, you don't even need a plate!

Most kids would agree that they like playing with their food! Temaki (tem-ack-ee) sushi, or hand roll sushi, is one of the most portable, fun, and delicious ways to enjoy sushi. Temaki sushi means "sushi in a cone." In this recipe, we demonstrate how to make your own plant-based sushi rolls. Of course we encourage your family to use any ingredients that you and your kids may love. Fish sticks? Chicken nuggets? Tofu? Cereal? Go for it. (Totally joking about the cereal. Just don't.)

You and your family can easily make sushi at home quickly and effortlessly. For our Temaki recipe, the biggest job is to prepare your fillings. I ask my kids to choose and chop up their favorite fruits and vegetables. Then you make the show-stopping sushi rice, get some nori sheets, pour the soy sauce, set up a buffet of ingredients, and BAM, you can have your own hand roll party. Anytime. Everyone makes their own! Once my family and I got the hang of Temaki, we were whipping up heaps of hand rolls in infinite flavor combinations.

My 3 daughters have so much fun patting the vinegared rice onto the nori, filling it with all kinds of delicious, healthy ingredients. Each one is unique. I adore watching my 12 year old daughter, Vivian, chow down tons of her favorite cucumber-avocado hand rolls, and I just smile knowing I am not shelling out the dough for sushi restaurant prices. The entertainment value alone of making temaki at home is priceless!

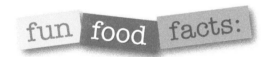

What does the word *sushi* really mean?

Sushi translates to "it's sour," and it refers to the lovely sweetly-vinegared rice, that alway accompanies sushi preparations. The main element is the rice. Sushi rice is typically topped or combined with nori (seaweed), a variety of vegetables, fruits, egg, fish and seafood.

Pop Quiz!

Sushi originated in Japan ...... TRUE or FALSE?

If you guessed "true," you're ...... wrong. WAIT, huh?!

Sushi was not invented in Japan. Over 600 years ago, rice and raw fish were fermented together to create a delicious, sour rice, in Southeast Asia. This method to create sour rice spread to China and then, eventually, to Japan. Today, sushi chefs added vinegar and sugar to cooked short grain rice to create that irresistible sourness (without all the fuss).

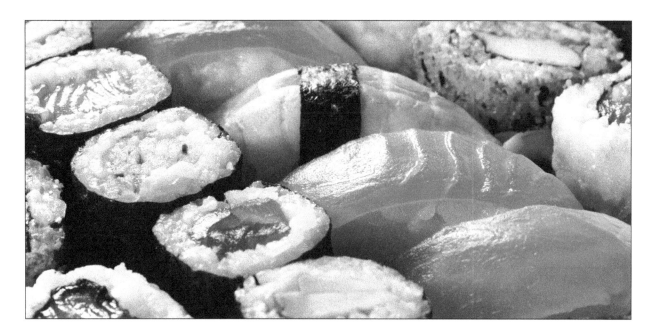

Where does sushi as we know it today come from? Sushi's popularity happened in the 1800's, when it became a fashionable and smart street food in Japan. Yes, there was fast-food even 200 years ago! A rice ball, vegetables, and (maybe) a sliver of raw fish requires very little preparation, it's easy to eat on the move, and it's a very delicious and healthy food choice.

What is *umami*? Um... a... what? After sweet, salty, bitter, and sour, the "fifth taste" that is recognized is Umami (ooh-maa-mee). Umami was identified by a Japanese scientist over 100 years ago. Yeah, science! Umami is usually described as a kind of a meaty, uniquely savory, and satisfying taste that is always abundantly present in sushi, nori, and in soy sauce.

How do you eat sushi? This is the best answer. YOUR HANDS! You're not supposed to use chopsticks. The traditional way to eat sushi is to hold the sushi piece with your fingers, kind of like it's a computer mouse. Then slowly flip the sushi over and lightly dip the side with the filling or toppings in the soy sauce. Try not to dunk the rice into the soy sauce (it's considered to be bad sushi etiquette).

What is *nori*?

You know the papery, dark green wrapping that keeps pieces of sushi neatly contained. Nori (naw-ree) is the Japanese name for edible seaweed. Some people might consider seaweed an unusual food, but it is a common item found in many of the world's kitchens and highly nutritious. Nori is a very ancient food that dates back nearly 3000 years. Originally, nori was only eaten as a ground up paste, which is still widely consumed today. The time of the Shoguns of Tokugawa, also known as the Edo period (1603 to 1868), was when nori we use today for sushi was invented through traditional Japanese paper-making techniques.

Nori is made by shredding edible seaweed, then pressing it into thin sheets, and letting it dry. Nearly exactly the same way we make paper. Nori that is sold as "plain" or "toasted" is the most versatile for sushi recipes. Crisp sheets of this mild-tasting sea vegetable last forever in your

You know the papery, dark green wrapping that keeps pieces of sushi neatly contained. Nori (NAW-ree) is the Japanese name for edible seaweed. Some people might consider seaweed an unusual food, but it is a commonly found in many of the world's kitchens and highly nutritious. Nori is an very ancient food that dates back nearly 3000 years. Originally, nori was only eaten as

★ Lots of vitamin B1 and B2—equivalent of a serving of meat.

★ Vitamins A, B1, B2, B6, niacin, and vitamin C.

★ 30-50% of protein per serving.

★ 8 calories - (4 calories per sheet).

★ Increased energy in your body.

★ Healthier skin, hair, and eyes.

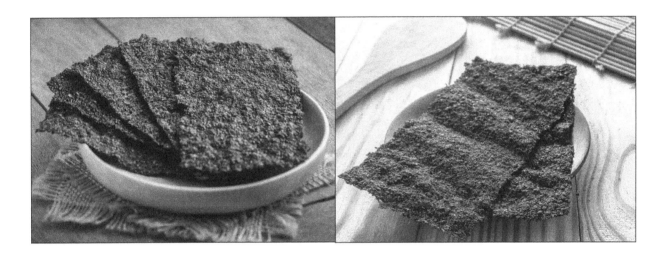

QUICK FACTS:

- Darker nori is the better nori. The darker the nori, the higher the quality.
- For thousands of years, nori has been a staple in many Asian diets.
- Common types of seaweed we eat are called nori, kombu, kelp, dulce, and Irish moss.
- Seaweed is a superpowered superfood.
- Seaweed can contain more protein than eggs, more calcium than cheese, and way more iron than beef.
- Seaweed helps prevent cholesterol from building up in our blood vessels.
- Seaweed is a very important and rich source of micronutrients (an abundance of essential nutrients)!

temaki sushi (hand roll)

hand roll ingredients

1½ C short-grain rice

¼ C rice wine vinegar

2 T agave nectar or sugar

1 tsp salt

8-12 nori seaweed sheets (large)

sushi roll fillings

choose at least 3, or as many as you want—feel free to make up your own with fruits + veggies:

cucumber

carrot

bell pepper

green onions

asparagus

cooked sweet potato

avocado

bean sprouts

tofu

apple

lettuce

snap peas

cooked mushrooms

green beans

cooked chicken

cooked fish

cooked beef

dipping sauce (ingredients to taste)

soy sauce

agave nectar or sugar

pre-step: cook the rice

In a colander, rinse **1½ cups of short-grain rice** with cool water until the water runs clear. Then let the rice sit to drain more the colander for 20 minutes. Place the rinsed, drained rice in a rice cooker (cook according to directions on your machine) or in a pot with a tight-fitting lid and add 3 cups of water.

Stove Method: Over medium heat, cover and bring the water to a boil. Boil for about 2 minutes, reduce heat and allow to simmer for another 5 minutes. Reduce heat to low and cook for about 15 minutes, or until water has been absorbed. Remove from the heat, remove lid, and place a towel over pot. Replace lid and let stand for 10 to 15 minutes. Do not refrigerate the rice. The rice will last up to 5 hours at room temperature without refrigeration.

important vinegar step: whisk+drizzle

Second to the rice, the most important sushi ingredient is the rice vinegar, which is really the soul of the sushi rice. The sugar and salt are added to flavor the sushi rice. Have your kids whisk together **1 tsp of salt, 2 T sugar or agave nectar** and ¼ **cup rice wine vinegar** in a bowl. Now have kids drizzle this seasoned vinegar you've just made over the pre-cooked rice and gently fold the vinegar into the rice by running a spatula through the rice in slicing motions to separate the grains. While doing this, slowly add the vinegar mixture. Add only as much as necessary; the rice should not be mushy. In Japan they fan the rice with an uchiwa (fan) during the cooling and mixing procedures. Have your kids fan the rice while you pour on the seasoned vinegar!

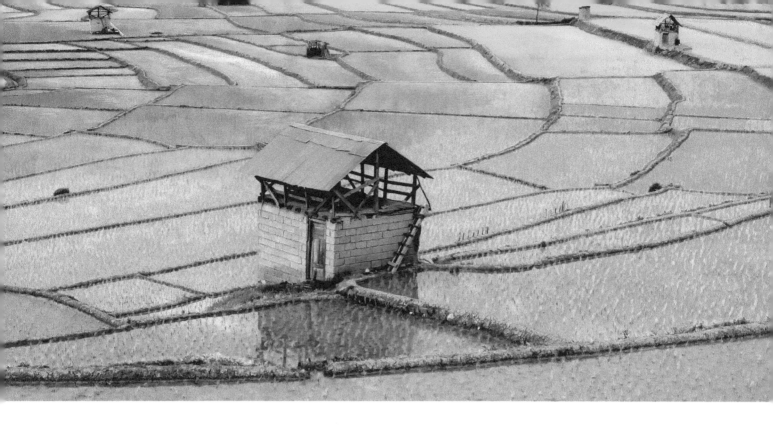

the fillings: slice+dice

Have kids slice and dice up the **tofu, fruits and/or vegetables** into matchstick-sized pieces. Sprinkle with a **little rice vinegar** as they chop and set everything on a plate in the middle of the table.

dipping sauce: pour+whisk

Now kids get to pour soy sauce and sugar or agave together until they agree on the taste. (We like a 4 to 1 soy sauce to sugar ratio.) Whisk and set to the side.

let's rock and roll them up-so let's: fill+fold+EAT!

(Refer to the following images for fun photo instructions!)

Have kids open up a large package of sushi nori. Then have kids cut the large nori sheets in half with scissors. Place a half sheet of nori horizontally in front of your child on a cutting mat. Place sushi rice on left third of nori (about 2 T of rice), leaving border of nori all around. Have your child child place whatever filling ingredients they choose vertically across middle of rice. Fold near corner of nori over to begin folding and rolling into cone shape. Continue to roll until cone is formed! It takes practice to roll sushi well, so don't worry if you don't get it right on the first try! (We sure didn't!) Just keep trying and keep in mind—even if they don't look so great, they will still be tasty! OISHII ("yummy" in Japanese)!

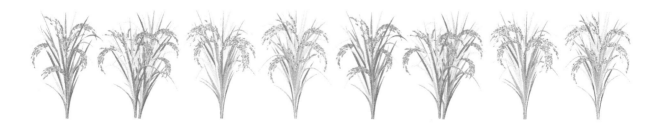

QUICK+EASY SUSHI STEP-BY-STEP!

Before you start, make sure your hands are dry in order to keep your nori dry and crispy.

Cut a large sheet of nori in half:

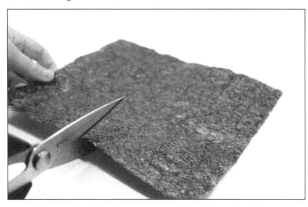 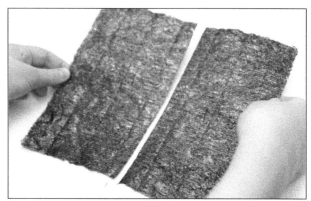

Place the <u>sheet of nori</u> on the palm of your hand (shiny side down) and put a thin layer of sushi rice on left third of the nori. Have your selected tasty fresh fillings handy.

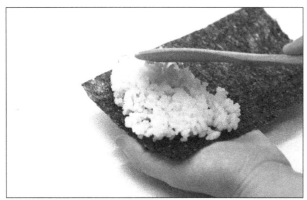 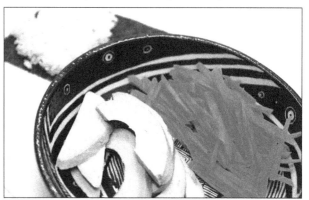

Place <u>fillings</u> vertically across middle of the rice.

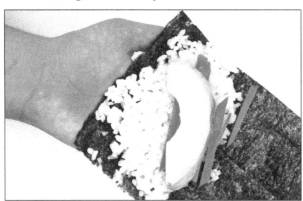

Fold the bottom left corner of nori over and begin folding into a cone.

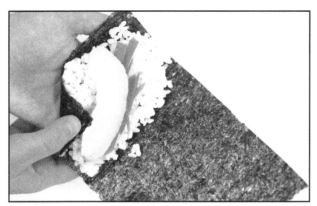 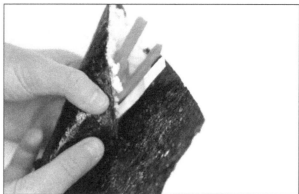

Keep rolling until cone is formed. You can put a piece of sushi rice at the bottom right corner to use as glue and close tightly.

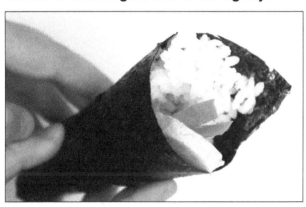

green tea soda

ingredients

3 bags decaf green tea bags
½ liter sparkling water
some ice

2 C hot water
sugar/agave/stevia to taste

snip+heat+sauté

Brew **3 decaf green tea bags** in **2 cups of hot water** and let steep for 5 minutes. Discard the tea bags. Add the brewed tea to your pitcher and stir in **sugar, agave or stevia (we used ¼ cups agave nectar)** to taste. Top the tea with **½ liter of sparkling water** and ice.

Stir and enjoy!

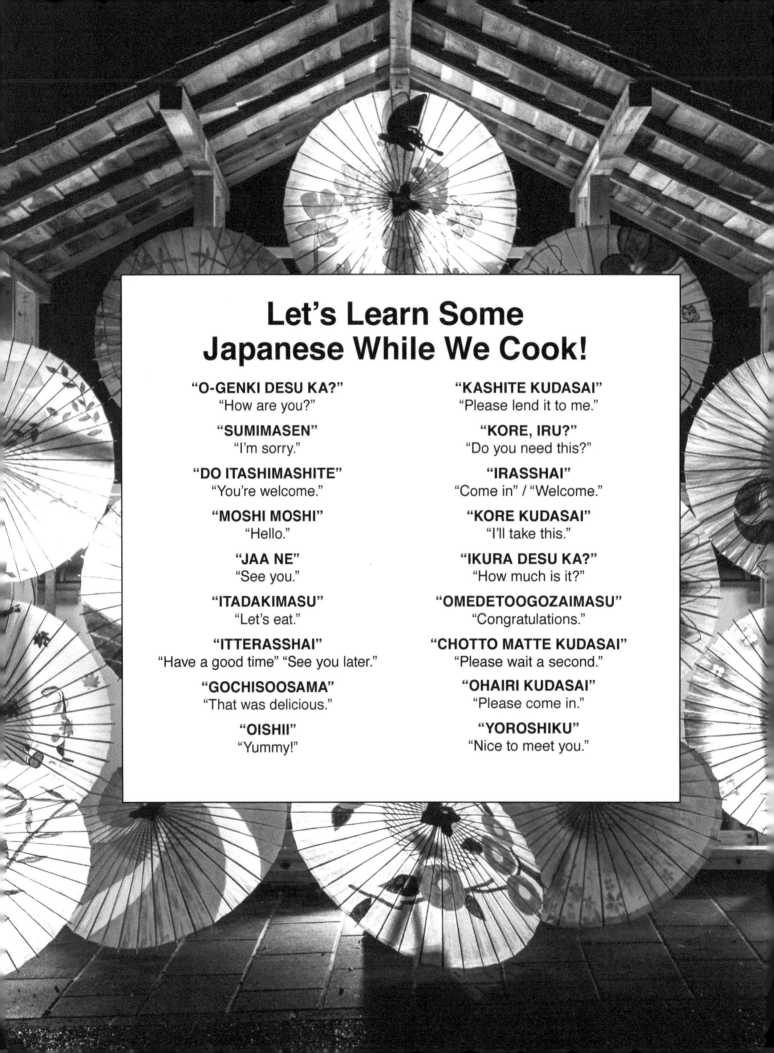

Let's Learn Some Japanese While We Cook!

"O-GENKI DESU KA?"
"How are you?"

"SUMIMASEN"
"I'm sorry."

"DO ITASHIMASHITE"
"You're welcome."

"MOSHI MOSHI"
"Hello."

"JAA NE"
"See you."

"ITADAKIMASU"
"Let's eat."

"ITTERASSHAI"
"Have a good time" "See you later."

"GOCHISOOSAMA"
"That was delicious."

"OISHII"
"Yummy!"

"KASHITE KUDASAI"
"Please lend it to me."

"KORE, IRU?"
"Do you need this?"

"IRASSHAI"
"Come in" / "Welcome."

"KORE KUDASAI"
"I'll take this."

"IKURA DESU KA?"
"How much is it?"

"OMEDETOOGOZAIMASU"
"Congratulations."

"CHOTTO MATTE KUDASAI"
"Please wait a second."

"OHAIRI KUDASAI"
"Please come in."

"YOROSHIKU"
"Nice to meet you."

Zany Stuffed Spring Rolls
+ Crispy Crazy Potstickers + Soy Ginger Drizzle + Ginger Hibiscus Punch

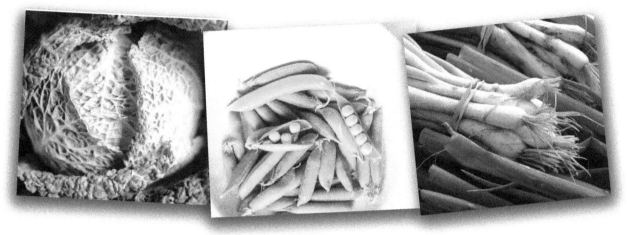

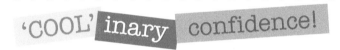

'COOL' inary confidence!

Cooking off the Cuff!

Have kid chefs choose their filling ingredients to add to the base of sautéed mushrooms, carrots, cabbage, and garlic! Let them choose how they're going to season their own dipping sauce. Also, have them wrap their wontons and spring rolls in different shapes. By giving kids creative liberty in the kitchen within a boundary of ingredients, they learn to explore and trust in their own ability to create delicious food!

Balancing Tastes! Chinese cooking is all about simplicity and using short cooking methods to bring out the best flavors of the ingredients used. Harmony is key in the final dish. Focus on texture, and a balance of sweet, salty, and sour tastes! Give kids the ingredients to choose from and let them decide how they're going to put them together!

Tools used in this recipe: Measuring Spoons, Dry Measuring Cups, Mixing Bowls, Liquid Measuring Cup, Whisk!

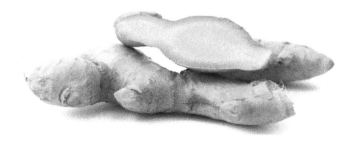

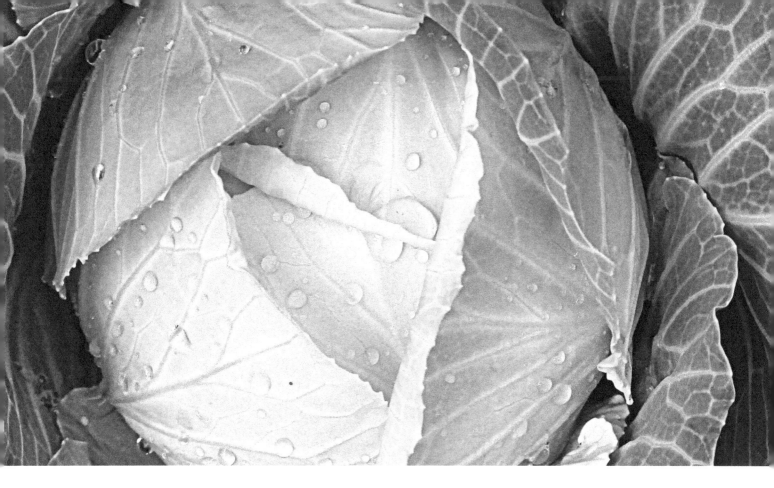

Surprise Ingredient Fact!

Cabbage is high in fiber, vitamin C, and vitamin K. Vitamin K is good for the blood. A cup of raw cabbage has more vitamin C than an orange!

Different varieties of cabbages have varying nutritional strengths: purple cabbage has more vitamin C, while Savoy cabbage has more vitamin A, calcium, iron, and potassium.

To Be a Kid in China!

Kids usually attend school from about 7:30 a.m. until 5 p.m. Students typically wear school uniforms, and their day starts with a morning exercise, after which their morning classes begin. They have a two-hour break for lunch in the middle of the day, followed by more afternoon classes.

There are many celebrations throughout the year in China that children attend—activities and celebrations to celebrate Chinese New Year, Spring Lantern lighting, and a Dragon Boat Festival every summer. For Chinese New Year, kids are often gifted with round objects, like oranges, coins, or other round-shaped sweets. An even number of gifts is traditional—such as 2 oranges instead of 3. Some kids receive money in red envelopes. Red is a color of good luck!

crispy crazy potstickers + zany stuffed spring rolls

ingredients

3 mushrooms
1 carrot
1 garlic clove
1 T sesame or olive oil
2 C shredded coleslaw mix
salt and pepper to taste
potsticker/wonton wrappers
spring roll wrappers
¼ C olive oil (for pan-frying)

additional veggies to choose from:
handful snow/snap peas
1/4 C canned, frozen, or fresh corn
½ small zucchini
2 green onions
canned water chestnuts
canned bamboo shoots
1/4 cup cooked lentils

rinse+chop+grate+slice

Rinse **3 mushrooms**, then chop them into tiny pieces! Use a box grater or food processor to grate **1 carrot** (with adult supervision!). Chop up **1 garlic clove**. Then slice or grate any other veggies you've chosen: **snow/snap peas**, **corn**, **zucchini**, **green onions**, and **water chestnuts**, **bamboo shoots,** and/or **lentils**.

sauté+season+mix

Heat **1 T sesame or olive oil** in a medium skillet and add chopped garlic, chopped mushrooms, and **2 C shredded coleslaw mix**. Sprinkle with **salt** and **pepper** and sauté until veggies are soft, about 3-4 minutes over medium heat. Then set aside this mixture to cool slightly. Mix in whatever other veggies you've chosen - have kids pick! Mix and match the fillings to make a few different options.

add+fold+seal

Set up a clean cutting board, a small bowl with water, the **potsticker** and **spring roll wrappers**, and the bowls of filling to get ready for assembling!

To make potstickers: Place a potsticker/wonton wrapper on the cutting board, then add 2 tsp filling to the middle. Trace the edges with a finger dipped in water, then fold up and seal into any shape you wish! Heat a non-stick pan over medium heat and add ¼ C of olive oil. Add the potstickers in the pan and fry for 2 minutes, without touching. Once the 2 minutes are up, gently add 1/3 cup water to the pan, turn the heat down to low, cover, and cook for another 2 minutes.

To make spring rolls: Place a spring roll wrapper like a diamond on the cutting board, then add 2 T filling just above the bottom corner of the wrapper. Roll up from the bottom corner until the filling is encased. Then fold over the sides toward the middle and continue rolling to the top!

panfry+steam+drizzle+eat

Adults: heat ¼ **cups olive oil** in the same skillet over low heat. Carefully add potstickers and spring rolls and panfry until one side of potstickers is golden brown and all sides of spring rolls are golden brown. Add **2 T water** to the skillet, cover it, and finish cooking by steaming for about 2-3 minutes. Remove potstickers and spring rolls from skillet and let cool slightly. Then drizzle with **Soy Ginger Drizzle** and ENJOY!

● ●

soy ginger drizzle

ingredients

1-inch piece ginger
2/3 C soy sauce/tamari/coconut aminos
2 T rice vinegar
2 tsp sugar or honey

1½ tsp sesame or olive oil
sesame seeds (optional)
green onion, sliced (optional)

peel+grate

Use the back of a plastic or metal spoon to carefully peel a **1-inch piece of ginger**. Adults: use a zester to grate the ginger (a box grater will also work and is a job best saved for you!)

measure+whisk+taste

Measure **2/3 C soy sauce/tamari/coconut aminos, 2 T rice vinegar, 2 tsp sugar or honey, 1½ tsp sesame or olive oil**, *small pinch grated ginger* and **1 T water** and add to a mixing bowl. Whisk to combine. Have kid chefs taste for balance! The sauce should be sweet, sour, and salty all at once. Add more of any ingredient to adjust. Then let kid chefs decide if they'd like to add **sesame seeds, sliced green onion,** or more grated ginger to the mix! Drizzle on pan-fried potstickers and spring rolls!

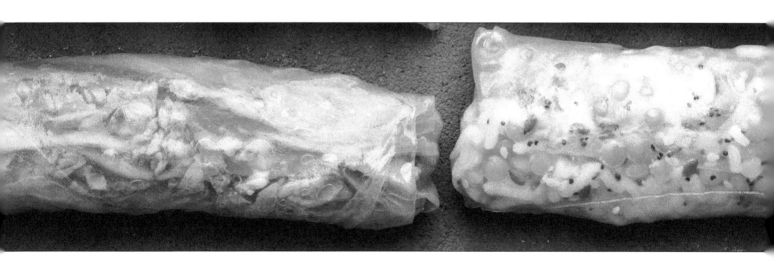

Italian Orange Carrot Polenta Zeppole
+ Quick Chocolate Orange Glaze + Candied Carrots + Italian Cocoa-Orange Lattes

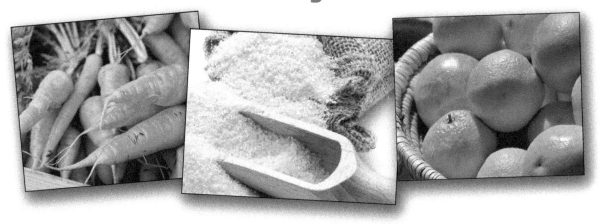

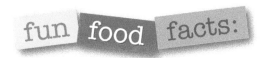

The History of Doughnuts!

Variations of doughnuts are found in every culture around the globe. Records show that the Dutch were making *olykoeks*, or "oil cakes," as early as the mid-19th century. These early doughnuts were simple balls of cake fried until golden brown. Because the center of the cake did not cook as fast as the outside, the cakes were sometimes stuffed with fruit, nuts, or other fillings that did not require cooking.

Hansen Gregory, an American ship captain, had another solution to the uncooked center of these early doughnuts. In 1847, he punched a hole in the center of the dough ball, increasing the surface area and exposure to the hot oil, and therefore eliminating the uncooked center.

Doughnut holes are the small spheres that are made from the dough taken from the center of ring doughnuts. Doughnut sellers saw this opportunity to market "holes" as a novelty.

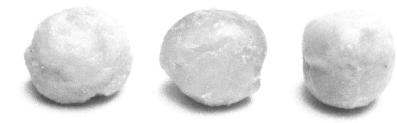

The featured ingredient: Oranges!

★ **Oranges are a great source of vitamin C, as well as dietary fiber.** Oranges are a good source of antioxidants. They also have about 8 grams of natural sugars per 100 grams of fruit.

★ **Oranges grow on trees.** The parent plant is spiny, small, and evergreen with glossy-green leaves and white fragrant flowers. During the first four years of its life, it bears very little fruit and it doesn't reach maturity until about 12 years old.

★ **Oranges can grow in a wide range of climates** but prefer warm temperatures as really cold weather can cause damage due to their small size and thin skin. In very hot weather, oranges can become sunburnt!

★ **Oranges must be picked carefully by hand when ripe.** They are difficult to harvest because their skins are easily bruised and damaged.

★ **Orange trees originated in China** and were later found in Europe. In the late 1400s, they were being grown in North America.

★ **The rind, or peel of an orange, is usually discarded, but can also be used in cooking.** The outer-most layer of the rind is called the zest and has a similar flavor to the inner part of the orange. The pith, or the white part on the underside of the rind, is almost always discarded as it has a bitter taste.

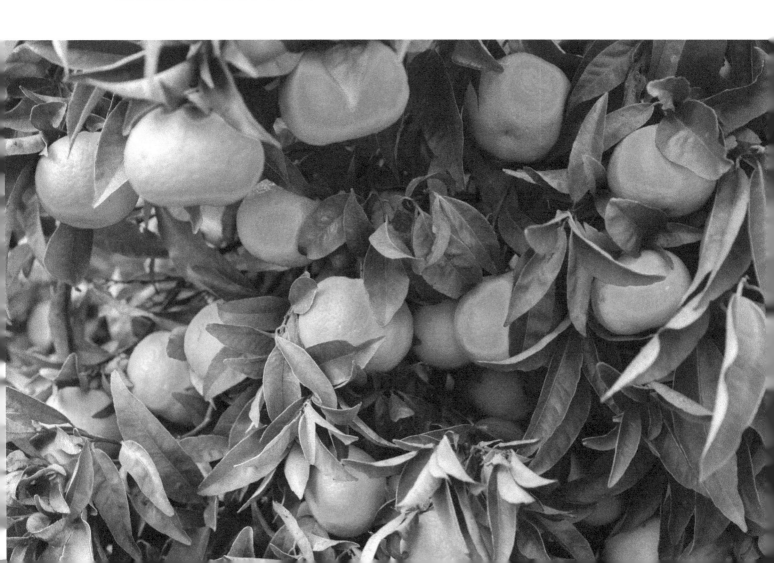

orange polenta zeppole doughnuts

ingredients

¼ C fine cornmeal

1¼ C water

¼ tsp + a pinch of salt

2 oranges (for ½ C juice + 1 T zest)

1 carrot

½ C (1 stick) butter

¼ C sugar

¾ C all-purpose flour

2 eggs

1 tsp vegetable oil

pre-cook+pre-heat

Combine **¼ C fine cornmeal** in a small saucepan with **1¼ C water** and a **pinch of salt**. Whisk until smooth while bringing to a boil over medium heat. Then continue to whisk for about 5 minutes until the cornmeal mixture has thickened. You have now made Polenta! YUM! Turn off the heat and let it cool. Preheat your oven to 400 degrees.

zest+squeeze+grate

Zest the rind of **2 oranges**. Squeeze the juice from the oranges after zesting. Grate **1 carrot**. This will be incorporated into the batter.

measure+combine+boil

In a skillet on your stovetop, combine **½ C (1 stick) butter**, **¼ tsp salt**, **¼ C sugar**, and **½ C freshly squeezed orange juice**. Bring to a boil over medium heat and then turn off the heat.

add+stir

Have your kids add **¾ C flour** and carefully stir into the melted butter mixture. Then add ½ C pre-cooked polenta and continue to stir everything together. If the dough is too wet, add more flour 1 T at a time to the skillet. Turn the heat back up to low and stir continuously until the mixture forms a ball, about 4 minutes. Transfer the dough to a medium bowl.

crack+blend

One at a time, crack **2 eggs** into the dough and blend with a hand mixer or an immersion blender —incorporating each egg completely before adding the next. Add 1 T orange zest and 2 T grated carrots to the dough and beat until smooth.

oil+bake

Time to make the zeppoles! Put **1 tsp vegetable oil** into each well of a mini muffin pan. Heat the empty muffin pan in the oven until hot. Then carefully pour in about 1 T of the batter into each cup.

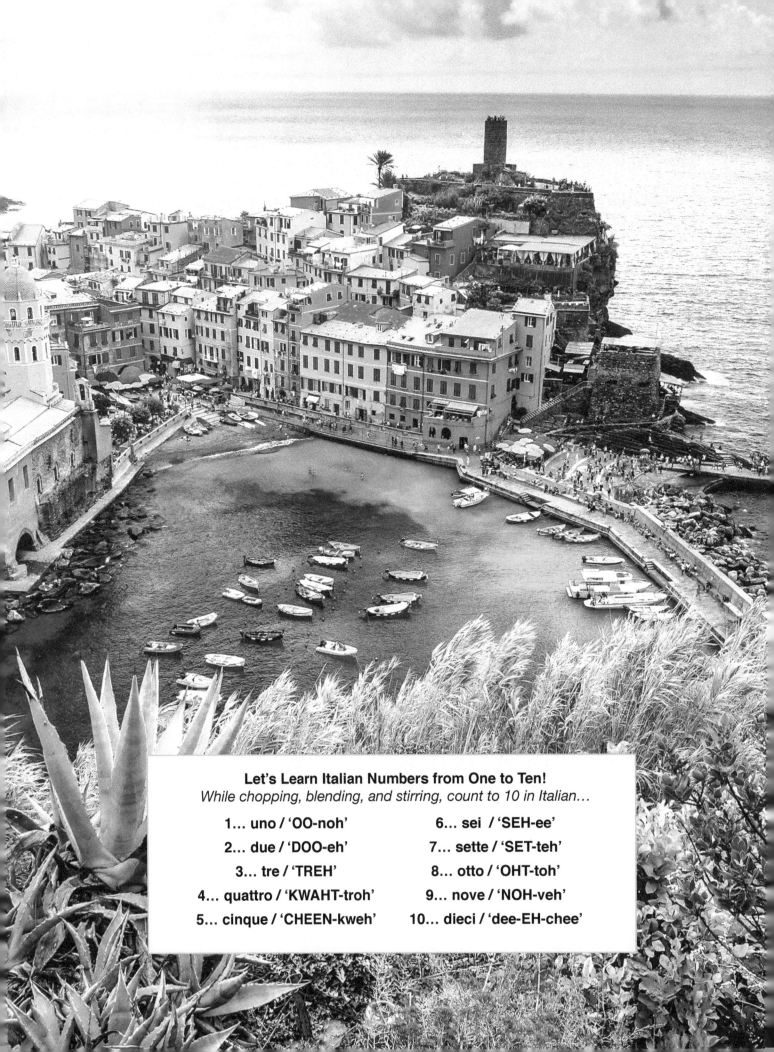

Let's Learn Italian Numbers from One to Ten!
While chopping, blending, and stirring, count to 10 in Italian…

1… uno / 'OO-noh'   6… sei / 'SEH-ee'

2… due / 'DOO-eh'   7… sette / 'SET-teh'

3… tre / 'TREH'   8… otto / 'OHT-toh'

4… quattro / 'KWAHT-troh'   9… nove / 'NOH-veh'

5… cinque / 'CHEEN-kweh'   10… dieci / 'dee-EH-chee'

candied carrots + quick chocolate glaze

ingredients

quick chocolate glaze
¾ C powdered sugar
2 T cocoa powder
1 T orange juice
pinch of salt

candied carrots
1 carrot
½ T sugar
1 tsp orange juice

grate+toss

Have your kids grate **1 carrot.** Toss the grated carrot with **a few drops of fresh orange juice** (to prevent browning) and **1 tsp sugar.** Set to the side while you make the glaze.

measure+whisk

Have your kids measure and whisk **1 T orange juice, ¾ cup powdered sugar, 2 T cocoa powder,** and **a pinch of salt** until smooth, creamy, and a little thick. Add more sugar if too thin and more orange juice (or water) if too thick!

squeeze+garnish

Squeeze the candied carrots dry with a paper towel. Top your zeppole with glaze and the candied carrots!

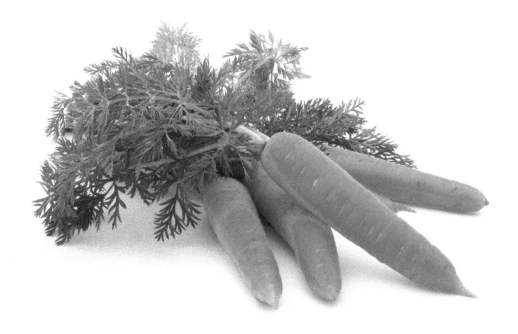

italian cocoa-orange lattes

ingredients

3 T cocoa powder

4 T sugar

peels of 1 fresh orange

3 C milk

combine+peel

In a small bowl, have your kids measure and stir together **3 T cocoa powder** and **4 T sugar** (or 2 packs Stevia) until well combined. Peel **1 orange**.

heat+stir

Heat **3 C milk** in a saucepan on your stovetop over medium low heat, with the orange peels. Stir in the chocolate/sugar mixture and heat until steaming. Let cool a bit and remove orange peels before serving!

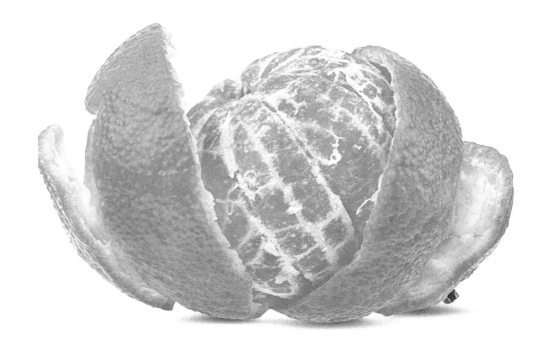

Fideuà Fantástico
(Spanish Noodle Paella)
+ Kid-Friendly Spanish Sangría

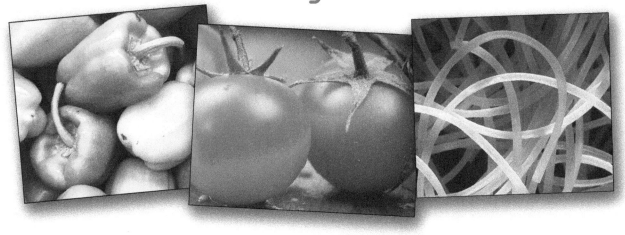

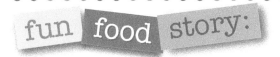

¡Esto es fideuà fantástico!

In 1997, my future husband and I sold all of our belongings to travel Europe together. We travelled wherever the wind blew us for 7 glorious months. We landed in Madrid, Spain and had our first taste of REAL paella. We were hooked. We asked the locals what region Paella was from and we were told to go to Valencia, Spain. We did. And spent 2 months eating paella. And drinking (way too much) Sangría.

I love the weather, the people, the rich history, and especially the food in Spain. My memories are vivid. Our 19-year-old daughter is now asking us to tell her stories about our life before she and her sisters were born. It is really fun for us to tell her about our wild, fun adventures together.

It also made me very hungry for our beloved paella. I wanted to have our daughters and our Sticky Fingers Cooking kids experience these lovely flavors, but being so busy in our lives, it needed to be quick and easy. I decided that Fideuà, paella's not so well-known "cousin," would fit the bill.

Fideuà is pronounced "feed de wa." This recipe is nearly the same as paella except for the main ingredient, which is fine pasta instead of rice. It is easy to make in a "snap," all in one pan. The kids LOVE breaking the noodles into small bits and helping with everything in the kitchen from step *uno* to *diez*.

This vegan version of a Fideuà, traditionally made with fish and shellfish, is loaded with good-for-you vegetables. I have revamped this traditional dish to make it easier to cook at home in any kitchen! Enjoy with some tapas, a fresh salad with fava beans, and our kid-friendly Spanish Sangría, and your family is ready for an authentic Spanish feast! You may even be able to remember those days, long ago, of letting the wind blow you from place to place…

Pura Vida (this is living!) Have fun + happy, healthy cooking! –Chef Erin

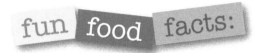

What the heck is Fideuà?

Fideuà is a cross between risotto and paella and is a dish for all lovers of Mediterranean fish soups in the bouillabaisse family. The chef and inventor was named Jan Bautista Pascual Sanchís. Better known by his nickname, Zabalo, this fisherman from from Gandia, Spain, near Valencia, first created the dish in 1930 at age 15. As the youngest member of the crew, Zabala was responsible for cooking and normally rustled up *arroz a banda*, rice cooked with fish stock. The problem was that the skipper of the boat ate more than his fair share, which left Zabalo and the rest of the crew hungry. Zabalo decided to use noodles instead of rice, thinking that the skipper may leave some more for them, but he ended up loving this version too!

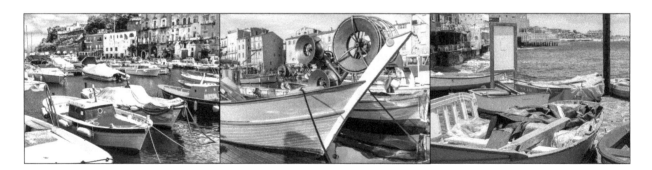

So fideuà was born and soon spread out of Gandia across the rest of the Valencia region of Spain and the rest of the world. In Catalunya, the northeastern part of Spain, there is a traditional dish called fideuà in which short lengths of dry pasta called *fideus* are cooked with a small amount of liquid in a wide, earthenware *cazuela* or paella pan, first browned in olive oil and then simmered in a rich fish and shellfish broth.

The featured ingredient: Bell Peppers!

★ **Bell peppers are actually fruits, not vegetables!**

★ **The most popular bell pepper in the United States is the green bell pepper.** Green and red bell peppers come from the same plant. As the bell peppers mature, their color changes from green to red as they ripen and become sweeter. That's why red peppers are sweeter than green peppers.

★ **Bell peppers come in all shapes, sizes, and colors!** Some are skinny and long while others are round or oblong. They come in all shades of red, green, yellow, and even purple and brown! They have a smooth, waxy skin and juicy, crunchy flesh.

★ **All bell peppers are rich in vitamin C,** but red peppers contain more than twice as much vitamin C as green bell peppers.

★ **Peppers are native** to Mexico, Central America, and northern South America.

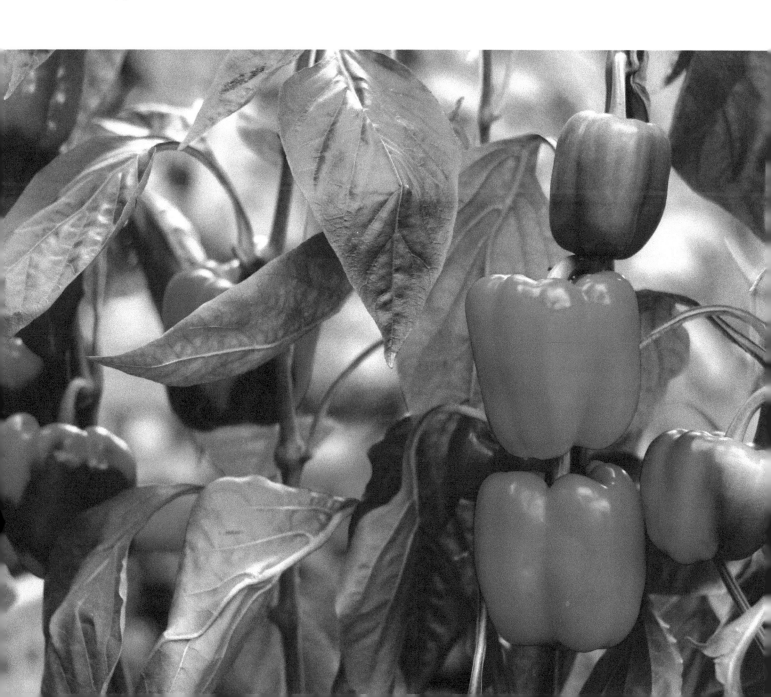

fideuà fantástico

ingredients

12-oz package thin spaghetti noodles

4 T extra virgin olive oil

2 cloves garlic

2-3 green onions

1 red bell pepper

1 green bell pepper

8 oz frozen peas

big pinch of salt

pinch of black pepper

½ T sweet paprika

28 oz can diced tomatoes

2 C vegetable broth

½ to 1 C canned garbanzo beans

1 lemon, sliced

break-up+toast

Place **12 oz uncooked thin spaghetti noodles** into a ziplock bag, seal, and have your kids break them into little bits. Then, in a skillet on your stovetop, add **4 T olive oil** and the broken noodles and toast until they are a deep golden brown. Watch the noodles carefully; you don't want them to burn!

chop+saute

Have your kids chop up **2 cloves of garlic**, **2-3 stalks of green onions**, **1 red bell pepper**, and **1 green bell pepper**. Add all of the chopped veggies, along with **1 cup (8 oz) frozen peas** and a **big pinch of salt** (to help get the moisture out) to the noodles. Sauté until the veggies are soft.

combine+simmer

Add a **pinch of black pepper** and ½ **T sweet paprika** and cook for 30 seconds. Then add one **28 oz can of diced tomatoes** (drained of all liquid), **2 C vegetable broth**, and ½ **to 1 C garbanzo beans**. Let simmer until noodles are tender. Do not stir. Cook for up to 15 minutes or until the pasta is al dente.

cover+rest

Turn the heat off the fideuà, cover with a lid, and let it "rest" for 5 minutes. Uncover and serve with lemon slices!

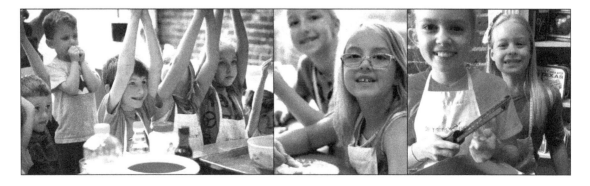

kid-friendly spanish sangría

ingredients

2 oranges
1 lemon
pineapple and/or apples and/or grapes
2 C juice (apple, cranberry, or grape)

4 C ginger ale
stevia or sugar to taste
ice

chop+throw

Have your kids chop up **2 whole oranges**, **1 whole lemon**, and other chosen fruit (**pineapple and/or apples and/or grapes**) and throw on the bottom of a large pitcher.

measure+stir

Have your kids measure **2 cups juice** (apple, cranberry, or grape), **4 C ginger ale**, and **2-4 C water** and pour over the fruit. Add **stevia or sugar**, to taste, and stir well. Add some ice last to hold the fruit down, and pour into cups, and drink up! Makes about 10 cups. *¡Olé!*

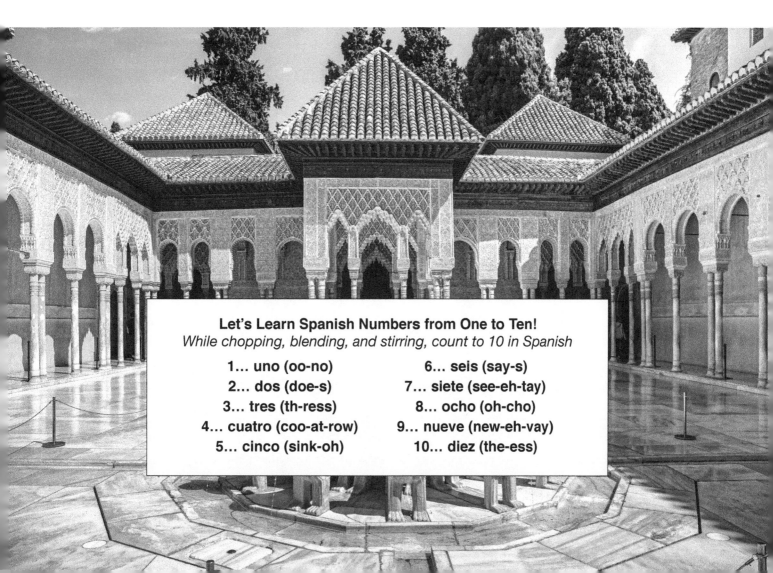

Let's Learn Spanish Numbers from One to Ten!
While chopping, blending, and stirring, count to 10 in Spanish

1... uno (oo-no)	6... seis (say-s)
2... dos (doe-s)	7... siete (see-eh-tay)
3... tres (th-ress)	8... ocho (oh-cho)
4... cuatro (coo-at-row)	9... nueve (new-eh-vay)
5... cinco (sink-oh)	10... diez (the-ess)

Greek Spanakopita Cups
Lettuce-Less Horiatiki Greek Salad + Green Greek Yogurt Shakes

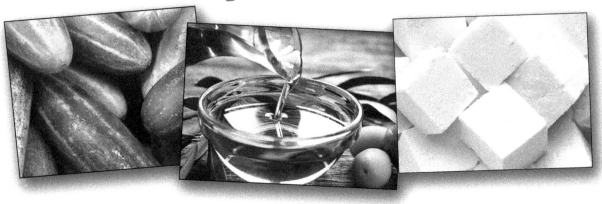

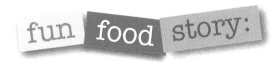

You're going WOW your kids with some delicious food from Greece with this recipe! Rustic, communal, colorful, and fresh, Greek food is one of our all-time favorites. We love its simplicity and purity. Greek recipes are wonderful because they encompass a pretty specific range of ingredients yet each dish stands apart on its own and is beautifully named, to boot.

Spanakopita (span-uh-KO-pee-tah) and horiatiki (hor-ee-AH-tee-kee) are two popular Greek dishes. Spanakopita is a traditional spinach pie made with phyllo dough. It is the perfect introduction to this rich culture of cuisine. We're turning the recipe into individual cups using wonton wrappers that are especially fun for kids to make!

Ask any kid (or adult) to name the main ingredient in salad, and what'll they say? Lettuce, probably. Traditional Greek salads typically don't have lettuce. *Horiatiki* translates to "village salad" and is typically made with an easy combination of farm-fresh tomatoes, cucumbers, red onion, olives, and olive oil—all things villagers always had on hand. To simplify things, we're making a straight cucumber Horiatiki with all the same seasonings of the original salad recipe, including oregano.

For our surprise ingredient, we're focusing on spinach! Why? Spinach is packed with nutrients, including chlorophyll, and is one of the milder, most versatile green leafy vegetables.

Spinach is also a main ingredient of spanakopita. Even our Greek Yogurt Shakes have a little spinach for extra nutrients and color. Enjoy cooking up these recipes with your kids, and don't forget to shout "Opa!" as you do. - *Happy + Healthy Cooking: Chef Erin & Chef Jacqui*

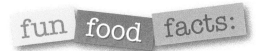

History of Spanakopita

We all know the word *pita*, as in pita bread. Well, in Greek *pita* means "pie." Who knew?! The English translation of Spanakopita = Spinach Pie.

This tasty dish may have originated over 400 years ago, and may have been introduced during the Turkish occupation of Greece. It is made with phyllo dough and commonly cut into triangles, and the interior is usually filled with cooked spinach and onions. For a heartier version of spanakopita, feta cheese is also added.

The triangular pastry can be made small, or in our Sticky Fingers Cooking classes, as a "cupcake," and it is to be served lukewarm, as is the traditional Greek way. One can purchase previously prepared spanakopita, ready for baking, to serve as appetizers or finger foods… but it is much more fun to make spanakopita yourself!

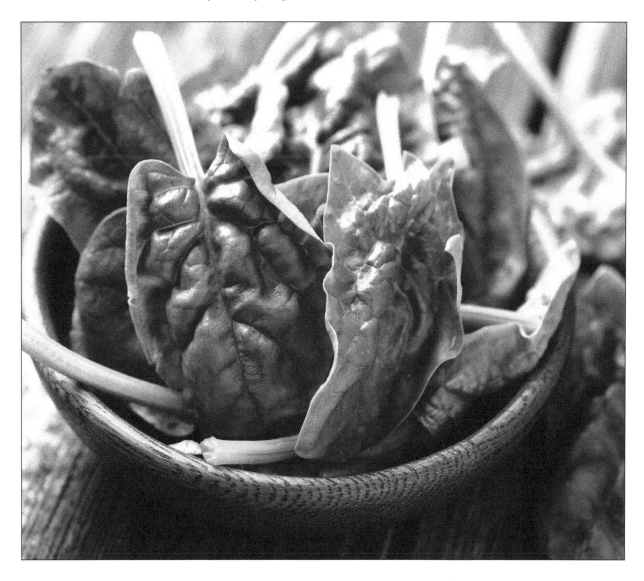

The featured ingredient: Spinach!

★ **Dark leafy green vegetables are some of the BEST foods we can feed our bodies.** Specifically, dark greens like spinach keep our hearts, blood, and brains healthy.

★ **Just half a cup of raw spinach counts as 1 of the 5-7 servings** of fruits and vegetables you should eat every day.

★ **Spinach is a source of vitamin K1,** which helps with blood clotting. How's this for interesting: Some French soldiers drank a mixture of spinach juice and wine during World War I to help recover after excessive bleeding!

★ **Spinach is high in chlorophyll.** In fact, all green vegetables (and plants) contain chlorophyll. Chlorophyll's job is to absorb sunlight and use it for energy - a process called photosynthesis. Chlorophyll helps the body create red blood cells and carry oxygen to our organs.

★ **Spinach can be eaten raw in salads and added raw to smoothies.** Spinach doesn't have a very strong taste, so it's a wonderful, fuss-free addition when you want to pack in more nutrition to whatever you're cooking. It can be chopped and added to soups and stir-fries, baked into gratins, quiches, and pies, pureed and added to dips. Frozen spinach is an easy substitute and works well in many recipes that call for fresh spinach.

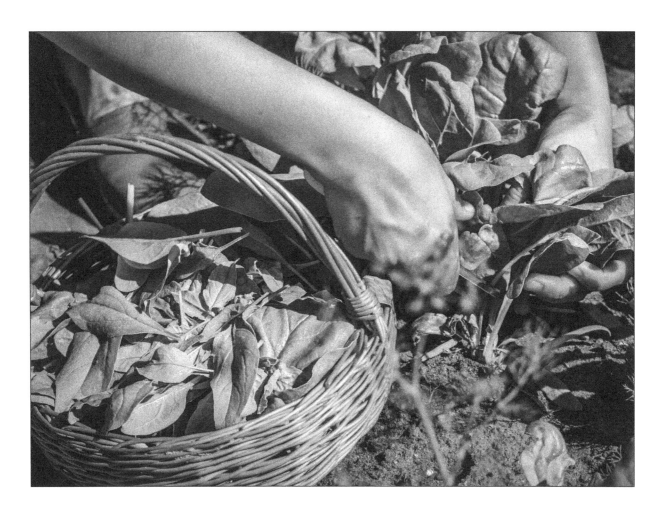

greek spanikopita cups

ingredients

5 oz frozen spinach, thawed
24 wonton wrappers
1 T olive oil
2 green onions
1 clove garlic
1 egg

½ tsp salt
pinch black pepper
4 oz feta cheese
1 tsp dried oregano
2 tsp brown sugar or honey
2 T plain Greek yogurt

preheat+squeeze+chop

Preheat oven to 400 degrees F. Place **5 oz frozen spinach** in a bowl and squeeze to remove the excess water. Set spinach aside and discard the water. (Reserve 1-2 T of the spinach for the green Greek yogurt shakes.) Then chop **2 green onions** and **1 garlic clove.**

sauté+crack+whisk

Heat **1 T olive oil** in a sauté pan and cook onions and garlic until soft (about 2-3 minutes). Meanwhile, crack **1 egg** in a bowl and whisk.

add+measure+mix

Add the sautéed onions and garlic to the spinach. Add the egg and **4 oz crumbled feta cheese.** Measure **1 tsp dried oregano, ½ tsp salt, a pinch of pepper, 2 tsp brown sugar or honey,** and **2 T plain Greek yogurt.** Mix well.

layer+bake

Take **2 wonton wrappers** and layer 1 tsp of spinach/feta mixture in the middle of the first wrapper. Then layer second wonton wrapper over that. Place 1 more tsp of spinach/feta mixture on top of the second wonton wrapper. Repeat with remaining wonton wrappers. Brush cupcake maker with oil, then place spanakopita cups in cupcake wells and press down so that they form to the wells. Bake for 8-10 minutes, or until spinach mixture has set and wonton wrappers are golden and crispy!

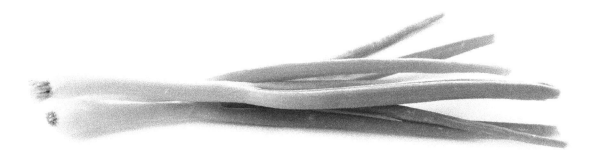

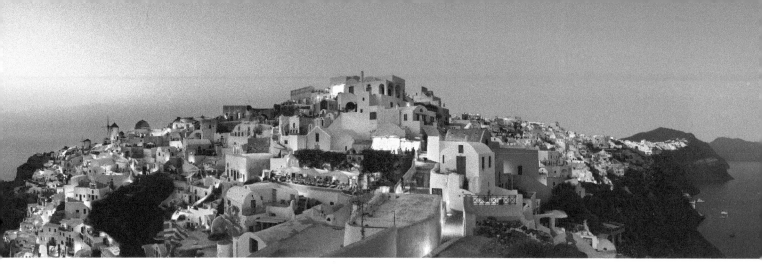

lettuce-less horiatiki greek salad

ingredients

2 cucumbers

1 lemon

1 T olive oil

1 tsp brown sugar or honey

½ tsp salt

½ tsp dried oregano

¼ cup crumbled feta cheese

dice+squeeze+whisk

Dice **2 cucumbers** into rough, chunky pieces. Squeeze the juice from **1 lemon** and whisk together with **1 T olive oil, 1 tsp brown sugar or honey,** ½ **tsp salt,** and ½ **tsp dried oregano.**

combine+toss+marinate

Combine diced cucumbers with salad dressing. Toss and let marinate for 20 minutes to allow flavors to meld. Just before serving, top with ¼ **cup crumbled feta cheese**.

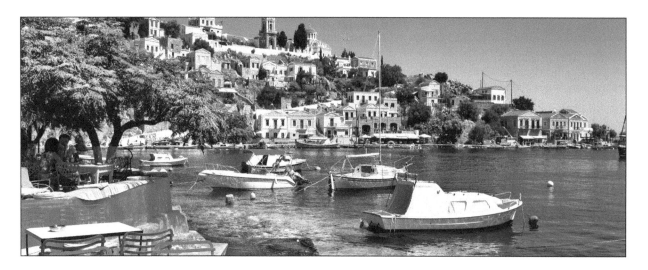

green greek yogurt shakes

ingredients

2 ripe bananas

1 C Greek yogurt

1-2 T frozen spinach

1 T brown sugar or honey

1 C ice

peel+add+measure

Peel **2 bananas** and add to a blender. Measure **1 C Greek yogurt**, a **handful of frozen spinach** (squeezed dry), **1 T brown sugar or honey**, and **1 C ice** and add to blender.

blend+pour

Blend on high until shake is thick and smooth (add a bit of water to help blend if needed!). Pour into cups and enjoy!

• •

cultivating 'cool'inary curiosity in kids ™

thyme for a fun activity

Yogurt Silly Putty Activity

Ingredients:

1 cup yogurt (no fruit chunks)

¾ cup cornstarch

Supplies:

mixing bowl

large spoon

directions:

- **In your mixing bowl, combine the yogurt and cornstarch** and mix to combine. Once the ingredients are loosely mixed, you might find it easier to switch to mixing with your hands.

- **When the mixture is no longer sticky,** pick it up and roll into a ball. If it's too sticky, sprinkle in more cornstarch. If it's too dry, add a bit more yogurt.

- **Enjoy the silly putty!** Make multiple batches if you have different flavors of yogurt. This putty does not store well - make a fresh batch to enjoy for the day!

Mini Finnish Mustikkapiirakka (Blueberry Pies)
+ Easy Peasy Lemon Drizzle +
Musikkamaito (Finnish Iced Milk)

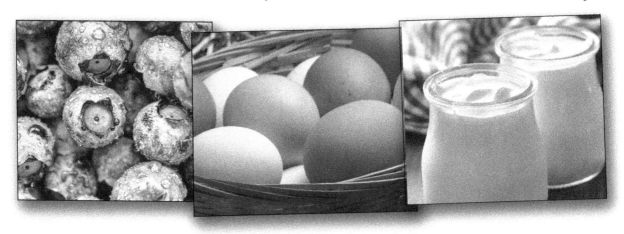

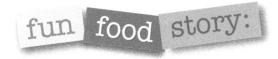

We cannot stop saying Mustikkapiirakka (MOO-STEE-Ka-PEEEEEE-Rah-Kah) at Sticky Fingers Cooking! It's really such a fun word!

Mustikkapiirakka is a traditional Finnish blueberry pie that we just KNOW your kids will have fun preparing and then savoring each mouthful when it is time to sit down to eat.

In the months of June and July, the entire country of Finland is cloaked in blueberries that grow wild. It's almost alarming if you've never seen it before. This traditional custard pie celebrates the seasonal bounty of blueberries. It's also very common in Finland to eat blueberries soaked in milk, especially when they're in season. This is a very simple recipe and remarkably delicious pie to bake at home.

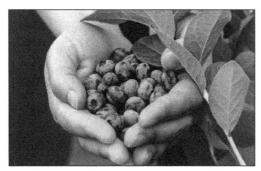
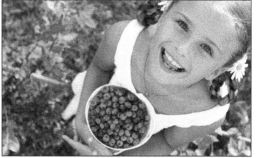

We became so excited about Mustikkapiirakka after coming across a home video on YouTube by Culinary Haven. All of us at Sticky Fingers Cooking would rather watch these humble videos from home cooks over fancy, overproduced cooking shows any day (and hope to get invited over someday for a slice of their Mustikkapiirakka pie!). *-Happy + Healthy Cooking: Chef Erin*

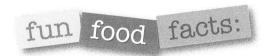

What is mustikkapiirakka?

Mustikkapiirakka is made by creating a sugary cookie-like crust and filing it with a delicious custard that is loaded with blueberries, baked until set, and then cooled a bit before eating!

As popular blueberries are in Finland, they are even more popular in the United States. You know the saying "As American as apple pie"? Well, no offense to the apple, but we would like to amend that saying: It should be "As American as *blueberry* pie" since blueberries are one of the few famous fruits to be native that are North America.

Blueberries are a big part of American history and culture. Native Americans realized the benefits of wild blueberries early on, utilizing their pleasant flavor and medicinal properties.

It wasn't until the late 1800s that people seriously tried to cultivate domestic blueberry bushes. At the turn of the century, a variety of highbush blueberries that yielded an abundance of fruit was cultivated. Today, 38 states grow blueberries commercially, 10 of which produce 98% of America's supply, making fresh blueberries available year-round so you can make you muffins, pancakes, and pies whenever you like!

The (not so) surprising surprise ingredient: Blueberries!

★ **Blueberries are one of the only natural foods that are truly blue in color.**

★ **Native Americans once called blueberries "star berries"** because the five points of blueberry blossoms make a star shape.

★ **The "bloom" of a blueberry refers to the pale, powder-like coating that protects the fruit.**

★ **Both Minnesota and New Jersey claim the blueberry muffin as their state muffin.**

★ **Blueberries contain a lot more antioxidants other fruits and vegetables.** Antioxidants may help prevent heart disease and cancer, and the anthocyanin present in blueberries is good for eyesight.

★ **A blueberry extract diet improves balance,** coordination, and short-term memory and is good for eyesight.

★ **Blueberries are one of the only natural foods that are truly blue in color.**

★ **Native Americans once called blueberries "star berries"** because the five points of blueberry blossoms make a star shape.

★ **The "bloom" of a blueberry refers to the pale, powder-like coating that protects the fruit.**

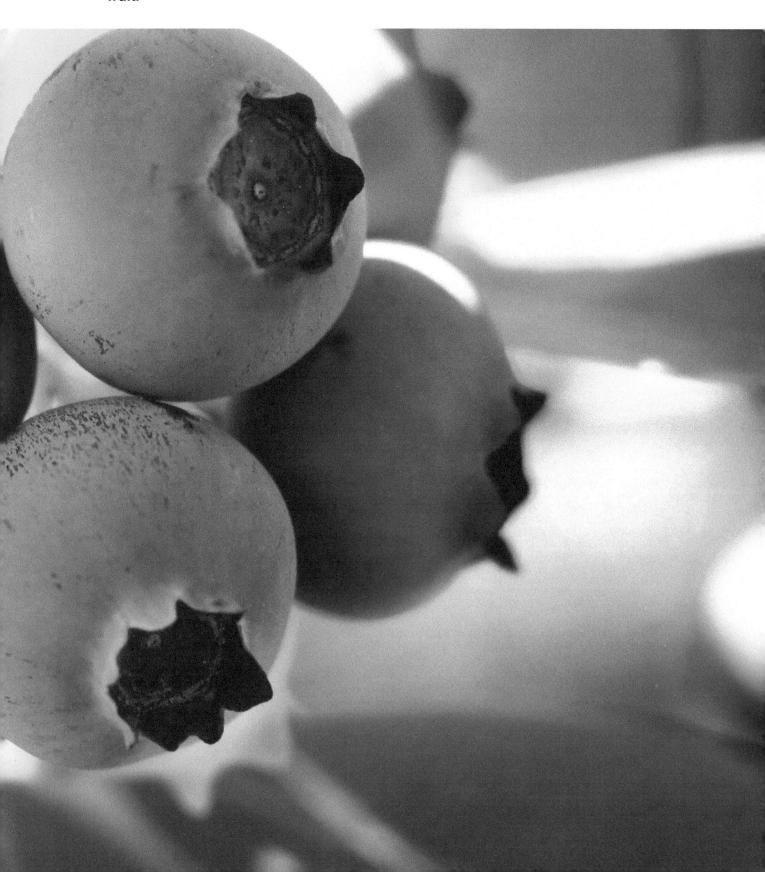

mini finnish mustikkapiirakka

ingredients

Pie crust ingredients:
1 C flour
¾ C sugar
¾ C softened butter
2 eggs
½ tsp baking powder

Pie custard ingredients:
1 C whole milk, plain Greek yogurt
1 tsp vanilla extract
2 eggs
¼ C sugar
1 C blueberries

measure+mix

Put the ¾ **C sugar,** ¾ **C softened butter,** and **2 eggs** into a large mixing bowl—and mix up everything with a fork. Next, measure **1 C of flour** and ½ **tsp baking powder** and add to the mixing bowl with sugar/butter/eggs. Now it is time to mix-up everything again until all is well combined.

press+bake

Press about **1 T of crust** into each well of a cupcake pan, spreading it out evenly. Then pop the tray into the oven for about 5-10 minutes until the crusts begin to get slightly golden. Then remove.

combine+stir+fold

Now it's time to make the pie custard! In a clean mixing bowl, combine **1 C whole milk, plain Greek yogurt, 1 tsp vanilla extract, 2 eggs,** and ¼ **C sugar.** Stir everything up and then gently fold in **1 C blueberries.**

spoon+bake+drizzle

Spoon about 1 T of pie custard into each mini pie crust in your cupcake tray. If there is any batter leftover, divide it equally amongt all the cupcake wells. Bake in your preheated oven until the custard is set, about 15-20 minutes. Drizzle easy peasy lemon drizzle over pies before serving!

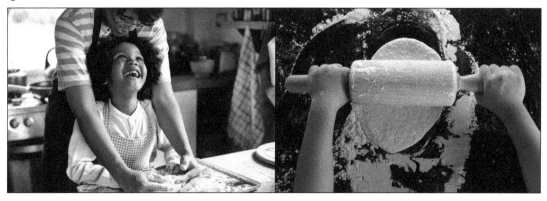

easy peasy lemon drizzle

ingredients

½ C powdered sugar

zest of 1 lemon

1 T lemon juice

zest+combine+dissolve

Zest **1 lemon** and combine lemon zest with ½ **C powdered sugar** in a mixing bowl. Then, add 1 T lemon juice and stir until powdered sugar has dissolved into the lemon juice.

adjust+drizzle

Adjust more lemon juice or more powdered sugar to get the perfect drizzle-able consistency! Drizzle over blueberry pies before serving!

blueberry musikkamaito

ingredients

½ C blueberries

2 C milk

2-3 T sugar (or 2 packs stevia)

1 C ice

measure+add+blend

Measure and add ½ **C blueberries**, **2 C milk**, **2-3 T sugar**, and **1 C ice** to your blender, or a pitcher for use with an immersion blender. Blend until creamy and thick. Taste and adjust flavors to your liking!

Let's Learn Finnish Numbers from One to Ten!
While chopping, blending, and stirring, count to 10 in Finnish

1... **yksi** (ook-si)

2... **kaksi** (cuck-si)

3... **kolme** (col-mey)

4... **neljä** (nell-yah)

5... **viisi** (vee-si)

6... **kuusi** (koo-si)

7... **seitsemän** (sates-eh-man)

8... **kahdeksan** (kah-deck-san)

9... **yhdeksän** (yuh-deck-san)

10... **kymmenen** (kumm-en-en)

Kid-Created Sweet and Savory Middle Eastern Hummus + Bite-Sized Dippers + Cinnamon Milk Tea

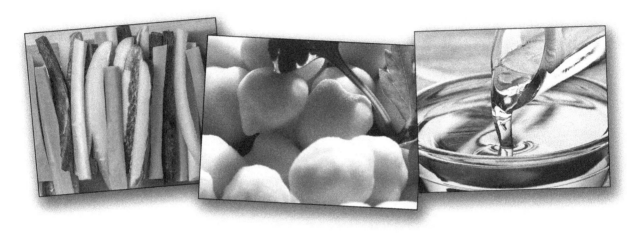

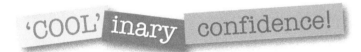

Cooking off the Cuff!

Have kid chefs choose their hummus add-ins for savory and sweet, jazzed-up versions of this classic recipe! Let them choose how they're going to season their hummus: Cinnamon sugar? Chocolate? Cinnamon? Chile powder? Lime? Also, encourage them to decide how they want their hummus to look. Chunky or blended or mashed? By giving kids creative liberty in the kitchen within a boundary of ingredients, they learn to explore and trust in their own ability to create delicious food!

Tools used in this recipe: Kid-friendly knives, cutting boards, hands, blender.

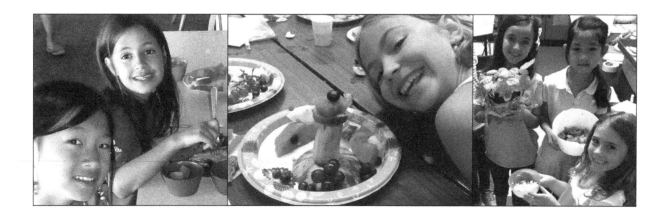

Foods of the Middle East and the Origins of Hummus!

The Middle Eastern region sits in Western Asia and Northern Africa and is bordered by the Mediterranean Sea. Seventeen separate countries make up the Middle East: Bahrain, Cyprus, Egypt, Iran, Iraq, Israel, Jordan, Kuwait, Lebanon, Oman, Palestine, Qatar, Saudi Arabia, Syria, Turkey, United Arab Emirates, and Yemen. The climate is HOT and DRY. People have been living there for thousands of years. Family is very important to the people of the Middle East.

Food culture is rich and varied, with many recipes and cooking methods overlapping. Middle Eastern art forms are stunning. Think handmade carpets, henna, marbling, glazed tile works, pottery, motifs, and embroidery.

Hummus likely originated in ancient Egypt! Though Greeks and Israelis also like to claim it as their own, historical records show that hummus was eaten in modern-day Cairo, the capital of Egypt, way back in the 13th century! That's over 800 years ago! Very classic hummus is made by boiling dried chickpeas and mashing with garlic, lemon, salt, olive oil, and tahini (a paste made from sesame seeds).

A typical meal in the Middle East is made up of meat, fish or a stew, and a sundry of vegetable dishes or salads. Meals are served with bread and/or rice, and often start off with a salad, appetizer, dip-like spreads such as hummus or baba ganoush, pickles and/or bowls of olives, dates, and nuts. Middle Eastern meals are FEASTS!

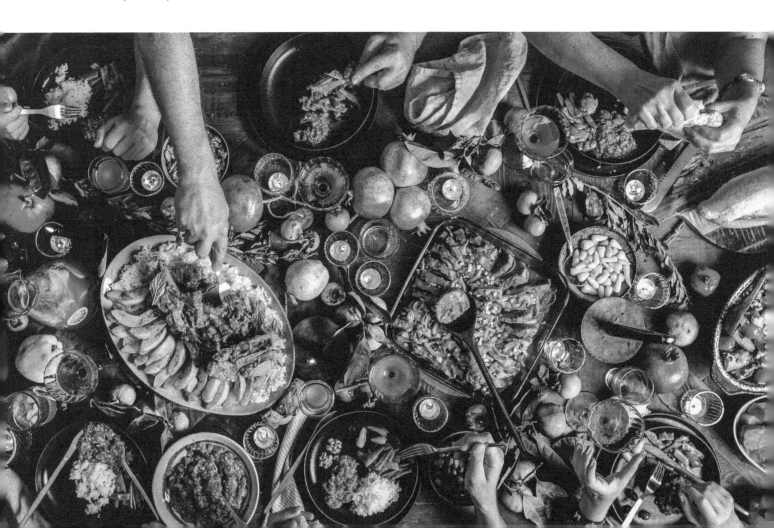

kid-created sweet and savory middle eastern hummus

ingredients

1 or 2 15-oz cans chickpeas
¼ C tahini

3 T olive oil

Savory add-ins:
minced garlic or garlic powder, lemon/lime zest or juice, salt, pepper, paprika, cumin, chile powder, oregano, basil, cilantro, etc.

Sweet add-ins:
cocoa powder, cinnamon, chocolate chips, mashed banana, canned pumpkin, sugar/honey/maple syrup, ginger, nutmeg, lemon juice or zest, etc.

measure+blend

Drain **1 or 2 15-oz cans of cooked chickpeas** (reserve the liquid!) and add to a blender or food processor. Measure and add **3 T olive oil** and **¼ cup tahini**. You could also make hummus out of frozen, thawed cauliflower, edamame, or canned (not pickled) beets! If the hummus is too thick, add a little bit of the reserved liquid and blend some more until you get the consistency you're looking for! Chunky or smooth!

season+mix

Scoop hummus into a bowl. To make sweet hummus, add any combination of the following ingredients: **mashed ripe banana, mashed canned pumpkin, chocolate chips, cocoa powder, cinnamon, nutmeg, ginger, lemon zest/juice and sugar/honey/maple syrup!** Taste as you go and have kiddos add more of any ingredient they choose. To make savory hummus, add any combination of the following ingredients: **fresh minced garlic** OR **garlic powder, lemon/lime zest or juice, salt, pepper, paprika, cumin, chile powder, oregano, basil, cilantro, etc.** Again, taste as you go and have kiddos add more of any ingredient they choose. Serve with Bite-Sized Dippers and Cinnamon Milk Tea!

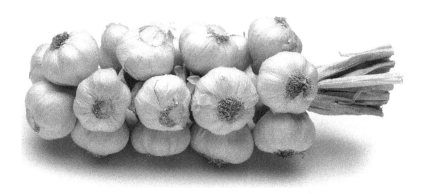

bite-sized dippers

ingredients

6 slices bread OR pita bread

olive oil

salt and pepper

1 cucumber

1 apple

2 stalks celery

1 red peper

handful baby carrots

slice+toss+toast

Slice **6 slices of bread** in thirds, then cut each third in half. If using **pita bread,** cut into bite-sized wedges! Toss sliced bread/pita with **olive oil** and pinches of **salt and pepper.** Heat a large skillet to medium, then toast bread until golden brown, flipping to toast both sides.

slice+chop

Slice **1 cucumber, 1 apple, 2 stalks celery,** and **1 red bell pepper** into bite-sized pieces. Arrange on a plate with a **handful of baby carrots**, toasted bread dippers, and serve with your delicious *Sweet and Savory Hummus!*

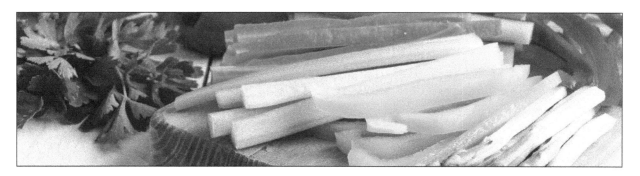

cinnamon milk tea

ingredients

2 C whole milk or milk alternative

¼ C sugar/honey/maple syrup

pinch of salt

big pinch cinnamon

measure+add+simmer+whisk

Measure and add **2 cups milk, 2 cups water, ¼ cup sugar/honey/maple syrup, a pinch of salt,** and a **big pinch of ground cinnamon** to a sauce pot. Bring to a simmer and whisk until sugar dissolves. Then pour into cups and CHEERS!

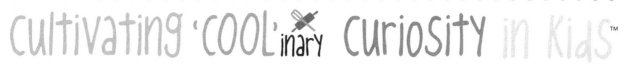
thyme for a fun activity

Magical Pepper Science Experiment

Ingredients:

handful of red pepper flakes
cup of water

drop of liquid dish soap

Supplies:

shallow tin or dish

Directions:

This quick observational experiment makes learning about surface tension and soap fun!

- **Fill a shallow tin or dish with about an inch of water.**

- **Before you sprinkle your pepper flakes into the water,** make a **hypothesis**, or an educated guess: What do you think will happen to the pepper when it hits the water? (The pepper should float - unlike salt, pepper is hydrophobic and does not dissolve in water. It does not sink either because water molecules—so tiny they're invisible to the naked eye—stick together and arrange themselves in a specific way that causes tension on the surface for certain things to float. Was your hypothesis right?

- **Now, squeeze a drop of liquid dish soap onto the counter and dip your finger into the soap.** You just need a tiny amount of soap.

- **Get ready to touch your finger to the surface of the water in the middle of the tin and make another hypothesis:** How do you think the pepper will react when soap touches the surface? (Woah! The pepper should dart to the edges of the tin when the soap comes into contact with the water. Since soap is such a powerful cleaner, it breaks down the surface tension of the water. But those tiny water molecules still want to do their job and maintain their surface tension, so they swim away from the soap. As they do that, the water molecules carry the pepper flakes with them!) Was your hypothesis correct?

- **For more fun, try repeating the experiment with different substances other than soap, such as hair spray or olive oil.**

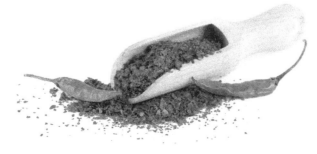

Turkish Apricot Garbanzo Olive Salad
+ Yufka Flatbread +
Turkish Delight Smoothie

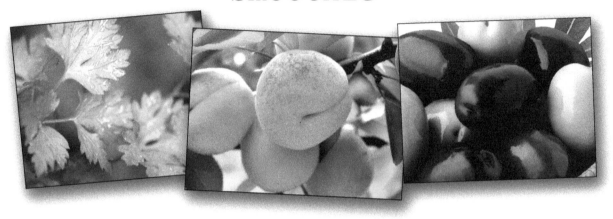

What is Yufka?

Yufka (yoof-KUH) is a type of Turkish bread. It is a thin, round, and unleavened flatbread. After kneading, the dough is allowed to rest for up to 30 minutes. The sheets of yufka dough are baked on a heated iron plate called a sac in Turkish. Baking time is approximately 2-3 minutes. During baking the bread is turned over once to brown the other side.

Yufka is a simple and delicious village bread. Normally it is cooked in an outdoor oven, but it works just as well cooked on a skillet. It is best served warm. One fun fact: the word *yufka* is also used as an adjective meaning "softie" or "tenderhearted," just like this soft bread!

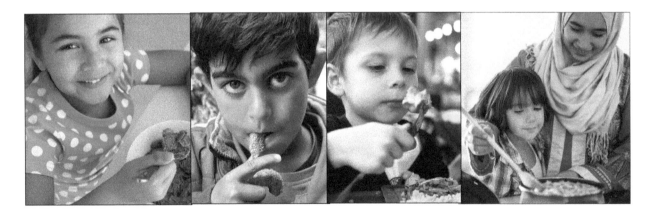

The featured ingredient: Apricots!

★ **Apricots were originally grown in China,** over 4000 years ago, and were brought to California by the Spanish in the late 18th century. California is the largest producer of apricots.

★ **Apricot pits have a hard shell because the seed inside is poisonous.** This keeps you from getting sick, while still allowing you to enjoy the healthy fruit!

★ **Apricots grow on trees, with peak season in June and July.** Since they have such a short season, over half of apricots grown are canned and many are dried.

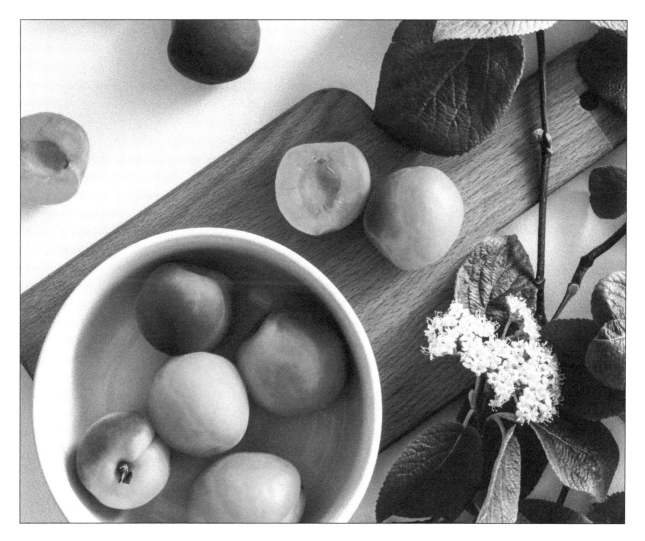

★ **Apricots are packed full of beta carotene, which becomes vitamin A in the body.** Vitamin A helps you see in the dark and makes your skin healthy. The deeper the orange color, the more beta carotene a food has, and the better it is for you.

★ **Apricots are also a healthy source of vitamin C,** which helps boost the immune system.

★ **Dried apricots are over 40% sugar,** so a little goes a long way in sweetening foods.

★ **Astronauts ate dried apricots on the Apollo moon missions.**

turkish apricot garbanzo olive salad

ingredients

15-oz can garbanzo beans, drained and rinsed
6 dried Turkish apricots
small handful fresh parsley
10 kalamata olives
2 T extra virgin olive oil

3½ T vinegar
1 large shallot
½ lemon, juiced
½ tsp salt
pinch black pepper
¼ tsp sugar or honey

chop+squeeze

Have your kids chop **1 large shallot** into tiny bits and add to a big bowl. Squeeze ½ **a fresh lemon** on top of the chopped shallots.

measure+whisk

In the bowl with the shallot, have your kids measure and whisk together **2 T extra virgin olive oil, 3½ T vinegar, ½ tsp salt, a pinch of black pepper,** and ¼ **tsp sugar or honey.** This is the dressing for the salad.

chop+tear+slice

Have your kids chop up **6 dried Turkish apricots** into small pieces. Next, tear up a **small handful of fresh parsley leaves,** and **slice up 10 kalamata olives**. Add everything to the salad dressing bowl.

add+toss

Add one **15-oz can of garbanzo beans** (drained and rinsed) on top of the apricots and olives. Toss the salad together and let it sit. The longer it sits the better. Before serving, taste it! Does it need more salt, vinegar, pepper, or sugar? Serve the salad at room temperature or even slightly warm.

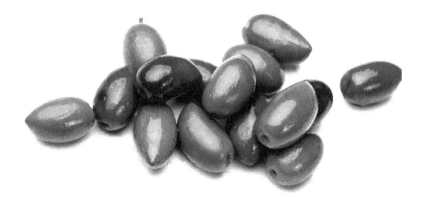

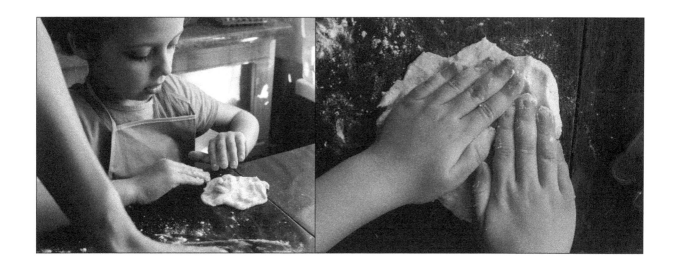

yufka flatbread

ingredients

2¼ C all-purpose flour

½ tsp fine sea salt

3 T olive oil

½ C warm water

2 tsp sugar or honey

salt, for sprinkling

stir+pour

In a large bowl, have your kids stir together **2 cups flour**, **½ tsp fine sea salt** and 2 tsp sugar or honey. Slowly pour **3 T olive oil** and **½ cup warm water**, while your kids simultaneously stir with clean fingertips in a circular motion. Continue to add enough water until the dough comes together.

knead+cover

Transfer the dough to a cutting board and have your kids continue to knead until it becomes soft and supple, about 3-5 minutes and up to 10 minutes. Cover with a damp kitchen towel and let rest for 5-20 minutes.

roll+shape+dunk

Have your kids roll and shape the dough into a 2-inch-thick log (like a snake!). Pinch off 12 golf ball-sized pieces and have your kids roll each piece in between their palms to form a smooth ball. Place about ¼ **cup flour** in a small bowl. Flatten each ball slightly and have your kids dunk the dough balls into the flour bowl. Finally, using a rolling pin or your hands, flatten each ball into a 6-inch-wide-ish circle.

cook+sprinkle

Heat a large nonstick or cast-iron skillet or griddle over medium heat with a little olive oil. Bake

stir+pour

In a large bowl, have your kids stir together **2 C flour** and **½ tsp fine sea salt.** Slowly pour **3 T olive oil** and **½ C warm water**, while your kids simultaneously stir with clean fingertips in a circular motion. Continue to add enough water until the dough comes together.

knead+cover

● ●

turkish delight smoothie

ingredients

2 C orange juice

1 large handful dried apricots

2 T sugar

10 ice cubes

1 banana

1 C yogurt

cinnamon and nutmeg

1 tsp vanilla extract

Combine+blend

Combine (in this order) **2 cups orange juice, 1 large handful dried apricots, 1 banana, 1 cup yogurt, 2 T sugar, 10 ice cubes, a dash each of cinnamon and nutmeg,** and **1 tsp vanilla extract** in a blender and blend until everything is well mixed, icy and smooth. Serve and enjoy!

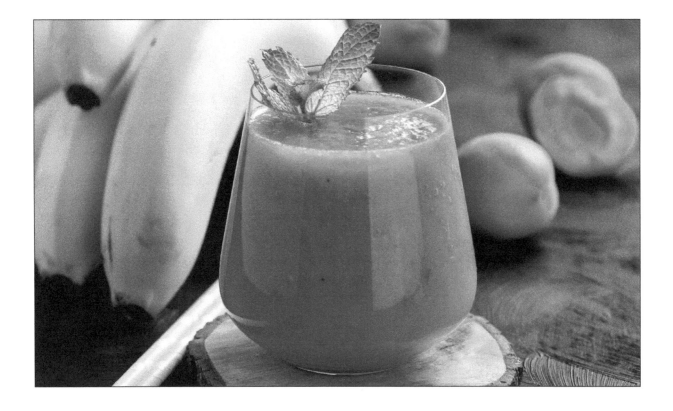

Fabulous Falafels
+ Cool as a Cucumber Dip +
Funny Flatbread

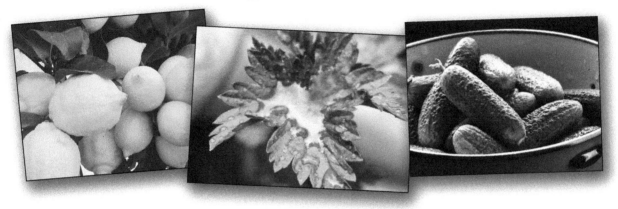

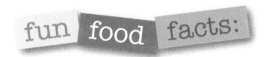 facts:

What is Falafel?

Falafel is a deep-fried ball or patty made from ground chickpeas and/or fava beans. It was first made in Egypt, though it has become a common form of quick and cheap street food and is often served as a *mezze* (appetizer) throughout the Middle East. Actually, falafel is often considered a national dish of Israel! Now, the hearty fritters are found around the world as a replacement for meat and as a form of tasty, quick street food.

★ **Garbanzo beans, also known as chickpeas,** Bengal grams, or Egyptian peas, have a delicious nutlike taste and buttery texture.

★ **Garbanzo beans originated in the Middle East,** the region of the world whose varied food cultures still heavily rely upon this high protein legume. The first record of garbanzo beans being consumed dates back about seven thousand years.

★ **The plant grows to be between 20 and 50 cm high** and has small feathery leaves on either side of the stem that grow white flowers with blue, violet, or pink veins. They grow seedpods containing two or three peas.

★ *Hummus* **is the Arabic word for "chickpea,"** called *garbanzo* in Spanish, *cici* in Italian, and *gram* in India.

★ **Garbanzo beans provide a concentrated source of protein** that can be enjoyed year-round are are available either canned or dried.

★ **The Latin name for garbanzo beans,** *Cicer arietinum*, **means "small ram,"** reflecting the unique shape of this legume that somewhat resembles a ram's head.

funny flatbread

ingredients

2 C all-purpose flour

1 tsp baking powder

1 tsp salt

1 C plain yogurt

olive oil

mix+stir

Have your kids mix together **2 cups flour, 1 tsp baking powder,** and **1 tsp salt.** Then, stir in **1 cup plain yogur**t until the dough is too stiff for a spoon.

knead+rest

Knead the dough in the bowl until it holds together well, adding more flour if necessary. Then turn the dough out on a floured surface and cut it into about 12 pieces. Have kids continue kneading the small dough balls for about 5 minutes, until the dough feels smooth and elastic. Put the dough balls in an oiled bowl, cover with a damp clean dish towel, and set aside to rest. Time to make the Falafels and the yogurt dip, then you can finish with the last step below!

press+oil+puff

Have your kids press the dough balls flat into round discs: the thinner the better, about ¼ inch or less is ideal! Brush some **olive oil** on a hot non-stick skillet on the stovetop and coat each dough disc with olive oil. Lay the dough discs on the hot skillet one at a time, fitting as many as you can on the skillet at once without overlapping, and cook over medium heat for about 2-3 minutes. It will puff up in places or all over, and there may be some blackish-brown spots on the bottom. Totally okay! Slide a spatula under the flatbread and flip it, and cook for a minute or two on the other side, just until it finishes puffing up into a balloon and begins to color lightly on top.

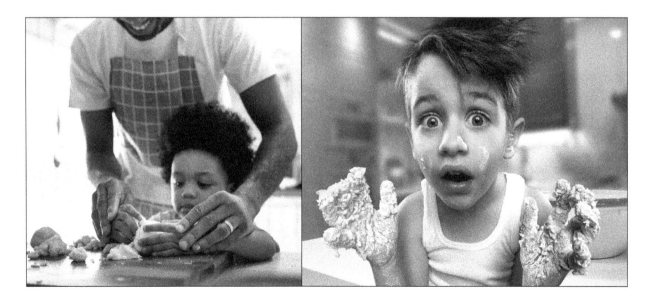

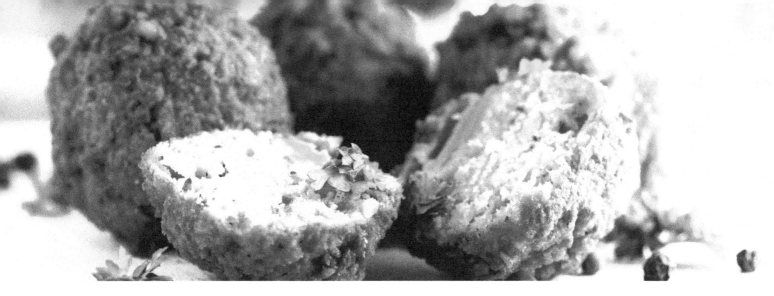

fabulous falafels

ingredients

2 15-oz cans garbanzo beans

2 tsp salt

1 tsp ground black pepper

2 tsp ground coriander

2 tsp ground cumin

4 T all-purpose flour

1 clove garlic

handful fresh parsley

1 lemon

½ small onion or 2 green onion stalks

pop+measure+toss

Have your kids "pop" the skin off of two **15-oz cans of garbanzo beans** (drained), discarding (or eating!) the skins. In a large bowl, combine the peeled garbanzo beans with **2 tsp salt, 1 tsp pepper, 2 tsp ground coriander,** and **2 tsp ground cumin.** Sprinkle **4 T flour** over the garbanzo bean mixture, toss together, and set to the side.

press+chop+squeeze

With a garlic press, squeeze **one clove garlic** into the garbanzo bean bowl. Chop up a handful of **fresh parsley, squeeze the juice of 1 lemon,** dice up **1 small onion,** and add to the bowl. Mix to combine well.

preheat+mash+roll

If baking, preheat your oven to 375 degrees and brush or rub a baking sheet with a thin layer of olive oil. (Stovetop instructions on next page.) Mash the garbanzo bean mixture with an immersion blender or food processor, making sure to mix ingredients together really well. You want the result to be a thick (yummy!) paste. Now have your kids roll the mixture into small balls, about the size of a ping pong ball. Slightly flatten the balls into a patty shape. Brush the tops of the falafel with some **olive oil.**

cook+enjoy

Either...

★ Bake for 20-30 minutes, gently flipping halfway through.

★ Cook on the stovetop (about 5 minutes per side) in a large oiled nonstick skillet or griddle over medium-high heat.

● ●

cool as a cucumber yogurt dip

ingredients

1 cucumber

1 green apple

handful parsley or mint

1 C plain yogurt

salt and pepper

grate+chop+tear

Using a cheese grater, have your kids grate **1 cucumber** into a large bowl, squeezing out the excess liquid with their hands and discarding it. Chop up **1 green apple** (with the skin on) into small chunks, then tear up a handful of **fresh mint or parsley** into small bits and add to the cucumber.

measure+whisk

Have your kids measure out **1 cup plain yogurt** and add to the cucumber mixture. Have kids take turns whisking the cucumber dip until smooth. Add **salt and pepper** to taste and serve with the falafels!

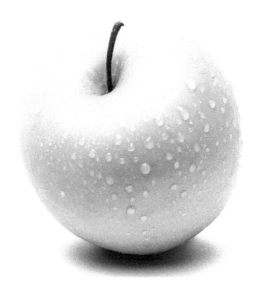

Real Rwandan
Spiced Honey Bread
+ Whipped Honey-Lemon Butter
+ Lemony Honeyed Milkshakes

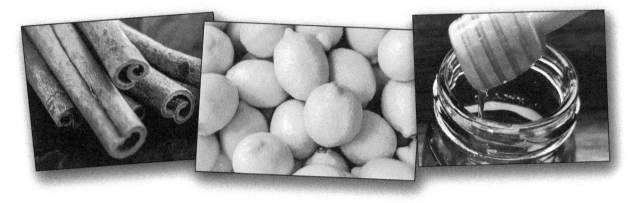

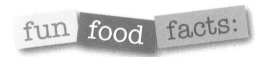

How does yeast work?

Yeast is the living organism that helps your favorite baked goods rise. The word *yeast* comes from the Sanskrit word *yas* which means "to boil or seethe." This ivory colored, single-cell fungus requires warmth, food, and moisture to work its magic.

Think about yeast like a dog—like a sweet little doggie named SEF (sugar eating fungus). Why? Well, a dog is alive and so is yeast. Of course, yeast is an organism and isn't going to jump up and snuggle with you, but it is alive and needs to be treated with care. A dog needs to be fed and so does yeast.

Yeast likes to eat sweet things like sugar or honey. Dogs need a bath and so does yeast. You don't want to give a dog too hot of a bath or you'll burn him, and the same is true of yeast. Dogs like to nap and so does yeast. Yeast needs time to rest and rise. Your dog burps and farts and so does yeast! This is the dog's and yeast's way of releasing gas.

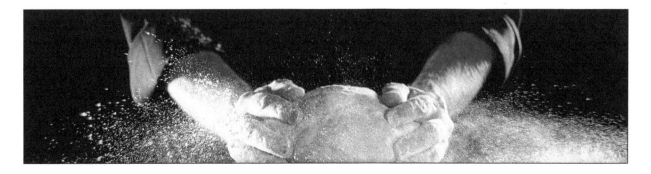

The featured ingredient: Honey!

★ **The word *honey* comes from the Hebrew language, meaning "enchant."** It is one of the oldest foods in the world. Honey is written about in hieroglyphics in caves.

★ **Honey is made by honey bees—the only insect in the world that make food that people can eat.** One bee will only make 1/2 tsp of honey in its entire life.

★ **Similar to how the Aztecs used cocoa beans as currency, the Egyptians valued honey in the same way.** Honey was fed to their sacred animals and also used as a tribute.

★ **Honey has an indefinite shelf life**—it can last forever if well stored because it has natural preservatives in it.

★ **Initially, honey was used to sweeten recipes, but now it is also used for its medicinal properties.** If you eat local honey (made from bees in the same area you live) regularly, you could build up a resistance to pollen thereby reducing your allergies. Honey can also help heal burns or cuts on your skin.

★ **Honey soaks up moisture quickly.** Try substituting half the sugar quantity with honey in your baked goods to keep them fresher and more moist for longer.

★ **There are many different types of honey,** which taste different depending on the flowers that bees collected nectar from to make it.

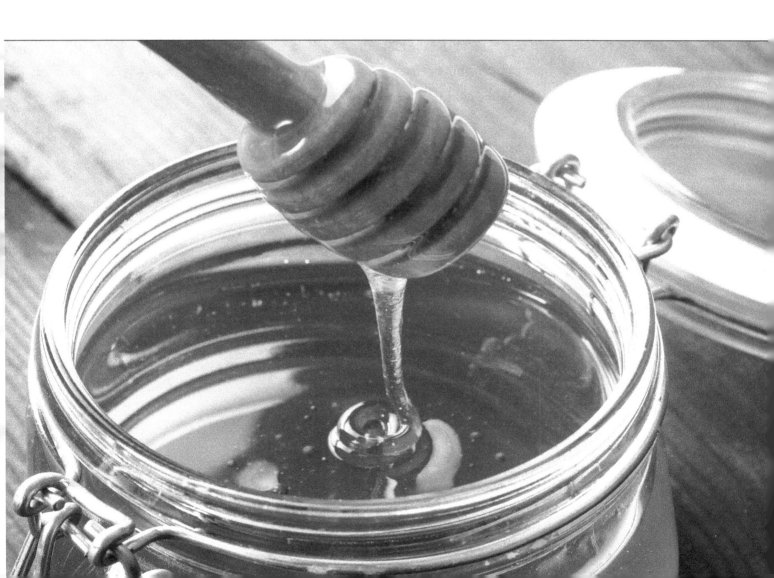

real rwandan spiced honey bread

ingredients

1 packet active dry yeast
3 C all-purpose flour + more for dusting
1 egg
½ C warm whole milk
½ C honey
¾ C lukewarm water

3 T vegetable oil
½ T ground coriander
¾ tsp ground cinnamon
¼ tsp ground cloves
¼ tsp salt

preheat+combine+rest

Preheat your oven to 375 degrees. Combine **1 packet active dry yeast** and ¾ **cup lukewarm water** in a large bowl. Let the yeast and water sit for 2-3 minutes. Stir and set aside to sit for another 10 minutes.

crack+whisk+mix

Crack **1 egg** into a large bowl. Then add ½ **cup honey,** ½ **T ground coriander,** ¾ **tsp ground cinnamon,** ¼ **tsp ground cloves,** and ¼ **tsp salt** and whisk everything together. Add ½ **cup warm whole milk, 3 T vegetable oil,** and your yeast and water mixture and mix again until well combined.

add+stir

Little by little, add **3 cups flour**, until the dough comes together. You want your dough to be soft, light, and not too wet, but you may not need all of your flour, so add it slowly. You may also need a bit more flour, so feel free to add as much as needed until the dough comes together.

knead+rest

Coat your hands in flour and turn the dough onto a floured surface. Knead the dough until it is smooth and springy. After about 5 minutes of kneading, set the dough in a clean bowl and cover it with a dish towel to let it rest for 10-20 minutes.

brush+roll+bake

Brush the wells of a muffin pan with oil. Pinch off 3 T of dough at a time, roll it by hand into a ball, and place into oiled cupcake wells. Bake for 15-20 minutes, or until the tops of the breads are golden brown and the dough has cooked through. Enjoy with a smear of whipped honey lemon butter!

whipped honey lemon butter

ingredients

½ pint (8 oz) whipping cream, room temperature
1 T honey

1 lemon
pinch of salt

zest+squeeze

Zest **1 lemon** and then cut the lemon in half and squeeze out the juice. Set both to the side. (You will use these in both the butter and milkshakes.)

pour+pinch+shake

Pour ½ **pint (8 oz) of room temperature heavy whipping cream** into a plastic container with a tight fitting lid. Add a **pinch of salt**. Cover tightly with a lid and then shake, shake, shake, shake until the cream becomes butter! When the cream stops moving in the container, you are almost there—keep shaking! When you hear a "clump and slosh," you have made butter!

drain+stir

Drain off the excess liquid (the buttermilk). Stir in a pinch of your lemon zest, a bit of your fresh squeezed lemon juice, and **1 T honey**.

lemony honeyed milkshakes

ingredients

½ pint (8 oz) heavy whipping cream
2 C milk
¼ C honey

juice of 3 lemons
2 tsp lemon zest
1 C ice

measure+combine

Measure and combine the juice of **3 lemons, 2 tsp lemon zest, 2 cup milk, ½ pint (8 oz) heavy whipping cream,** and ¼ **cup honey** to your blender or a pitcher, for use with an immersion blender.

blend+add+blend

Blend until well combined and then add **1 cup ice** and continue to blend until nice and smooth.

Corny Veggie
Mac 'n Cheese Cups
+ Crispy Veggie Streusel Crust
+ Classic Pink
Lemonade

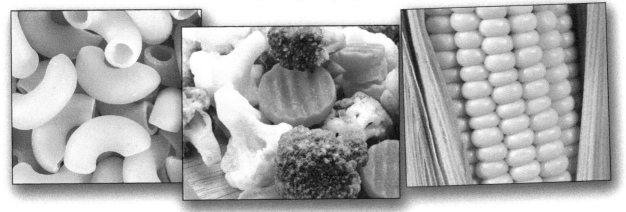

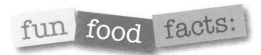

Let's learn about Corn!

Corn was first cultivated by indigenous people in Southern Mexico anywhere from 7.000 to 10,000 years ago.

Corn is unique: most vegetables and fruits we eat today are domesticated versions of wild plants humans discovered long ago. Corn is a human invention and did not exist in the wild first, although it DID start from a wild grass called teosinte. Teosinte didn't look how modern corn on the cob looks today. The kernels were much smaller and further apart.

Corn is produced on every continent in the world except Antarctica! Corn and cornmeal are staple foods of many regions.

Corn comes in many colors, including black, blue-gray, purple, green, red, white and yellow.

Corn is not technically a vegetable. It's a grass! As food, it's considered a whole grain. Popcorn is also considered a fruit. That's right! This is because fruit, like popcorn, comes from the seed or flower part of the plant.

Corn contains phosphorus, which is a mineral the body uses to build strong bones. Phosphorus also helps the body produce energy. Starches in corn also provide you with long-lasting energy.

Fresh corn on the cob is seasonal during the months of July and August. Avoid any corn that has dark or dried spots. Frozen corn is a great alternative when fresh corn isn't in season.

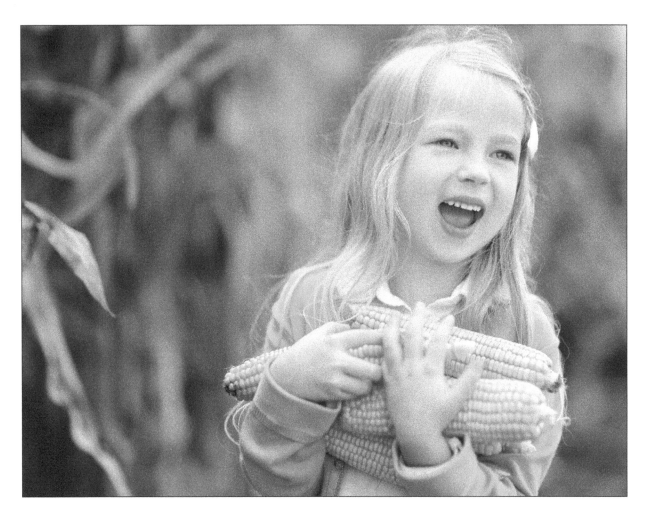

A Brief History of Mac 'n Cheese!

How did macaroni and cheese become such a popular American dish? One popular story says our 3rd American president, Thomas Jefferson, encountered macaroni and cheese for himself when he traveled to Paris and northern Italy in the 1700s.

He drew a sketch of the pasta and took detailed notes on how to make it. He brought the recipe back to the US. At that time, macaroni and cheese was considered a cuisine of the upper-class when he served it at stately dinners.

Thomas Jefferson had slaves who cooked for him, his family, and their guests. This explains why Mac 'n Cheese became and remains such a staple Southern Soul Food dish. During the Great Depression in the US in the 1930s, KRAFT invented a box version of macaroni and cheese. Mac 'n Cheese was now affordable and accessible to all Americans, and it's been a staple American dish ever since.

corny veggie mac 'n cheese

ingredients

1 C uncooked macaroni

2½ tsp salt

¾ C mixed raw veggies (broccoli, cauliflower, carrots, tomatoes, sweet potato, parsnip, etc.)

1 glove garlic

¼ tsp ground nutmeg

¼ tsp garlic/onion powder

¼ tsp ground pepper

¼ C heavy cream

1½ C grated cheese

¾ C frozen corn

preheat+soak+chop+mince

Preheat oven to 350 degrees F. In a medium-sized pot or large mixing bowl, soak **1 C uncooked macaroni** or other small shaped pasta noodles in 3 C warm water + **2 tsp salt** for 10-20 minutes. Chop **your choice of veggies** to total about 1½ C (reserve ½ C for the Crispy Veggie Streusel Crust (recipe below). Chop all veggies to tiny pieces! OR, if using parsnip or sweet potato, grate them. Mince **1 clove peeled garlic.**

step+step+step

Crack and whisk **2 eggs** in a mixing bowl. Using a grater, grate **2 T butter**. Add butter to the eggs, then measure and mix in ¼ **tsp ground nutmeg**, ¼ **tsp garlic/onion powder**, ½ **tsp salt**, ¼ **tsp black pepper**, ¼ **C heavy cream**, 1½ **C grated cheese** and the *minced garlic*. Add the *drained pasta*, ¾ **C frozen corn** and ¾ C of the minced veggies and mix again.

scoop+sprinkle+bake

Use an ice cream scoop to portion the Mac 'n Cheese into a greased muffin tin. Sprinkle with Crispy Veggie Streusel Crust. Bake for about 20-25 minutes, or until cheese has melted and is golden brown on top. Enjoy!

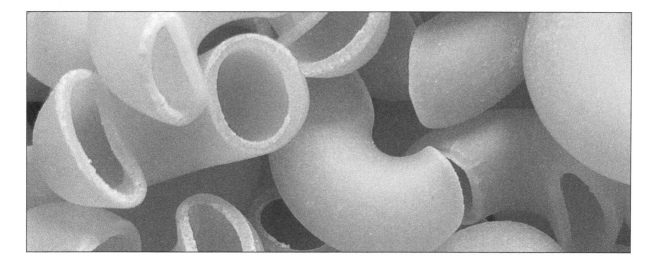

crispy veggie streusel crust

ingredients

½ C minced veggies

¼ C Italian or Panko breadcrumbs

¼ C all-purpose flour

2 T butter

pinch of salt

mix+sprinkle

In a mixing bowl, add ½ **cup minced veggies, ¼ cup Italian or Panko breadcrumbs, ¼ cup flour, 2 T butter,** and **a pinch of salt.** Mix with hands until a crumbly texture forms. Sprinkle evenly over Mac 'n Cheese Cups just before baking.

To make a dairy-free version, substitute 2 T olive oil for butter.

classic pink lemonade

ingredients

3 lemons

1 C cranberry juice

½ C sugar

Squeeze juice from **3 lemons** into a pitcher. Add **2 C cold water, 1 C cranberry juice,** and ½ **cup sugar.** Mix until sugar is dissolved, then pour over ice and enjoy!

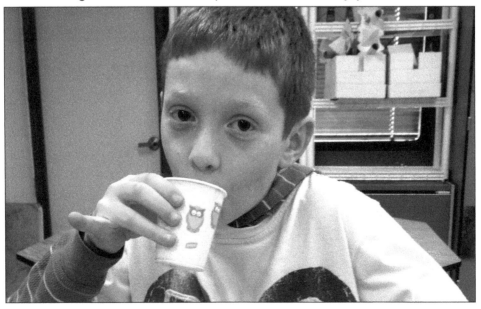

Kid-Innovated
Totally Tasty Tostadas
+ Speedy Skillet Refried Beans
+ Mexican Chili Limeade

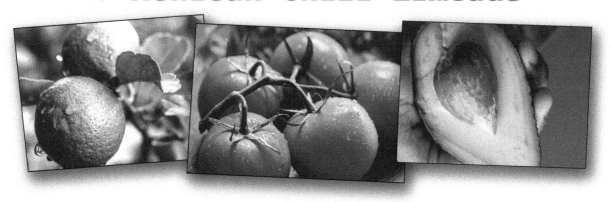

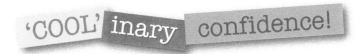

Cooking off the Cuff!

Have kid chefs choose their Tostada Toppings and encourage them to get creative with layering their final creations. Tostadas were invented to make use of tortillas that weren't quite fresh enough to be used for tacos but were still good enough to eat. Typically eaten whole, tostadas start with a layer of refried beans followed by more layers of chopped toppings, which may include either fish, meat, or even fried grasshoppers (in Oaxaca, especially!).

When kids have creative liberty in the kitchen within a boundary of ingredients, they learn to explore and trust in their own ability to create delicious food!

Tools used in these recipes: Kid-friendly knives, cutting boards, hands, blender, box grater, wooden spoon or potato masher.

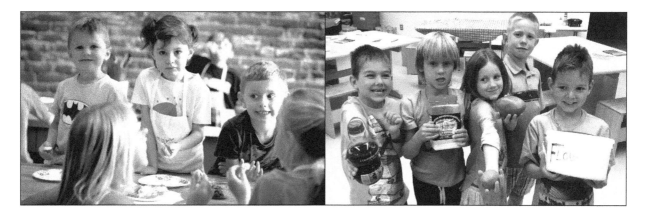

Food and Culture of Mexico: Fun Facts

★ **In Spanish, the word tostada means "toasted."** Tostadas are eaten in Mexico and other parts of Latin America.

★ **Pinto beans got their name from the Spanish word pintado,** which means "painted."

★ **Beans have B-vitamins!** High levels of vitamin B are excellent for the heart and brain: they improve brain function and memory.

★ **It is mandatory for kids to attend elementary school in Mexico.** Many children are homeschooled, especially in rural parts of Mexico.

★ **Children in Mexico often live with extended family**, such as cousins, grandparents, aunts, and uncles.

★ **15% of children in Mexico are working by the time they are 12 years old.** Working at an early age helps the extended families that often live together.

★ **Children in Mexico usually have two last names!** The first part of their last name comes from their father's first surname, and the second part comes from the mother's first surname.

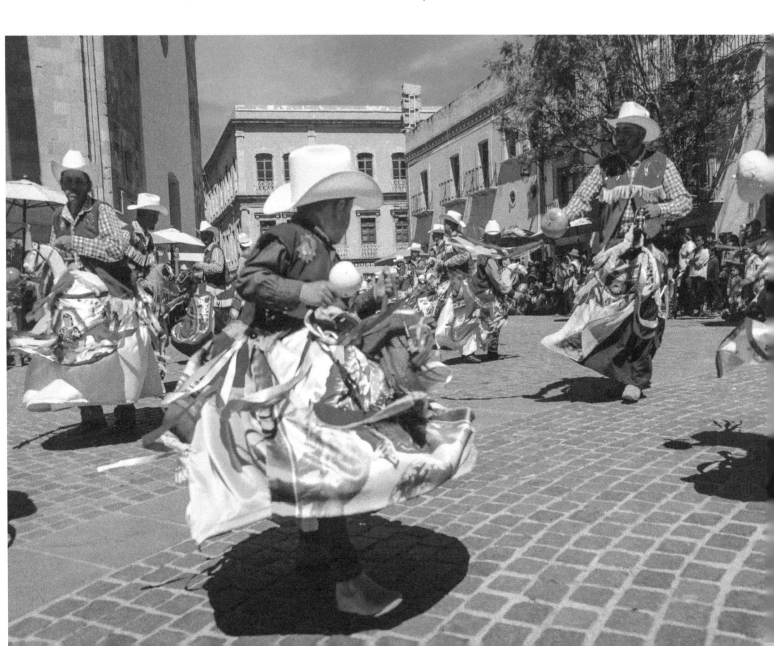

speedy skillet 'refried' beans + totally tasty tostadas

ingredients

2 big cloves fresh garlic
4 green onions
2 T olive oil
15-oz can pinto beans
½ tsp ground cumin
1 tsp salt
1 T butter
6 oz cherry tomatoes
1 bunch red radishes
½ head iceberg lettuce

2 large carrots
1 ripe avocado
½ can black olives
handful fresh cilantro
1 lime
1 pack tostada shells or tortilla chips
6-oz shredded Monterrey Jack or Cotija or Queso Fresco cheese
small container sour cream

mince+slice+sauté+cool

Have kids peel and mince **2 big cloves of garlic**. Thinly slice or cut with scissors **4 green onions**. Add **2 T olive oil** to a medium skillet and sauté the minced garlic and sliced green onions for a minute. Then add **15 oz can pinto beans** (dump the whole can in without draining it). Season with ½ **tsp ground cumin** and **1 tsp salt**. Sauté for 3-5 minutes. Turn off heat, then stir in **1 T butter** until it melts and let beans cool slightly.

mash+taste+season

Once the beans have cooled a bit (they can be warm, but not hot), transfer them to a mixing bowl and have kids mash them with the back of a wooden spoon or a potato masher until they're creamy and smooth. Take a taste and add more salt, or cumin if you want!

chop+slice+grate

Chop up **6 oz cherry tomatoes** and **1 bunch red radishes**. Thinly slice ½ **head iceberg lettuce**. With help from an adult, carefully grate **2 large carrots** using a box grater. Adults: Cut **1 avocado** in half, remove the pit, and slice the flesh of each halve thinly before scooping out the slices from the shell. Slice ½ **can black olives**. Chop or tear up the leaves of a **handful fresh cilantro**. Slice **1 lime** into squeezable wedges.

spread+top

To assemble tostadas: Spread a layer of refried beans onto each tostada. Top with **6-oz shredded Monterrey Jack or Cotija or Queso Fresco cheese,** and kids' choice of shredded lettuce, chopped tomatoes, shredded carrot, radishes, black olives, shredded cheese, and sour cream. It's fun to let kids decide how they're going to build their own tostadas!

mexican chili limeade

ingredients

4-5 limes

¼ to ½ C sugar

Pinch of salt

¼ tsp mild chili powder

squeeze+add+blend

Squeeze the juice from **4-5 limes** into a blender. Add **¼ to ½ cup sugar**, **4 cups cold water**, a **pinch of salt**, and **¼ tsp mild chili powder**. Blend until smooth and frothy. Pour into cups and *¡SALUD!* ("Cheers!" in Spanish)!

Let's Learn Some Spanish While We Cook!

Hello
¡Hola!
(Say: OH-la)

How are you?
¿Cómo está usted?
(KOH-moh ehs-TA oos-TEHD)

I am fine
Estoy bien
(ehs-TOY bee-EHN)

Please
Por favor
(pour fah-VOR)

Thank you
Gracias
(GRA-see-ahs)

You're welcome
De nada
(deh NA-da)

See you later
Hasta luego
(AHS-ta looEH-go)

Goodbye
Adiós
(ah-dee-OHS)

Nice to meet you
Mucho gusto
(MOO-choh GOOS-toh)

Yummy
Sabroso
(Sah-BROH-so)

Cuban Banana
Dulce de Leche Pancakes
+ Vegan Dulce de Leche Sauce +
Banana Dulce de Leche
Smoothies

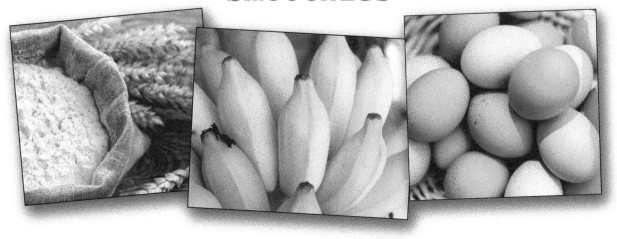

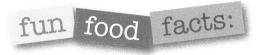

The History of Dulce de Leche (Caramel)

The word caramel was first recorded in the English language in 1725. It comes from the Spanish Dulce de Leche and Caramelo. The original Spanish word did not refer to the chewy caramel candy, but more likely, to caramelized sugar. Caramel candy and sauce were invented in the USA!

Caramel is simply sugar melted into a syrup and cooked until the sugar crystals turn into a dark amber liquid. In this form, it can be thickened into a sauce, turned into a frosting or filling, and used to coat nuts (pralines) and popcorn, to name a few. Whisk in some butter, remove from the heat before whisking in cream, and you have a delicious caramel sauce.

In fact, Milton Hershey began his chocolate empire not with chocolate, but with caramel. In 1886, he founded the Lancaster Caramel Company, utilizing traditional recipes found in many cookbooks. He chose to learn all about chocolate-making because he sought new coatings for his famous caramels.

cuban banana dulce de leche pancakes

ingredients

1¼ C all-purpose flour

2 tsp baking powder

big pinch sea salt

2 semi-ripe bananas

1 cup of your favorite milk

1 tsp vanilla

½ T light brown sugar

4 T butter, room temperature

1 large egg

measure+add

Have kids measure **1¼ cups flour, 2 tsp baking powder**, a **BIG pinch of sea salt** into a big bowl. (This is the dry bowl.)

chop+slice

Ask kids to peel, slice, and chop **2 semi-ripe bananas** into TINY BITS! Set to the side.

crack+stir

Have kids stir together **1 cup of your favorite milk**, **1 tsp vanilla**, **1½ T of light brown sugar** with **2 T room temperature butter** into a small bowl. (This is the wet bowl.) Show your child how to crack open **1 large egg**. Add the egg to wet bowl and mix together.

combine+mix

Have kids combine the wet ingredients into the dry ingredient bowl. Add the chopped bananas to the batter and mix well. Preheat your skillet to medium/low heat and melt about 2 T of butter.

spoon+flip

Spoon batter onto preheated skillet, forming small-sized pancakes. Cook out for about 2 minutes per side or until golden brown and bubbly. Flip over and cook the other side until golden brown and puffed.

top+yum

Transfer to oven-safe plate to keep warm in your oven and then serve topped with Vegan Dulce de Leche Sauce!

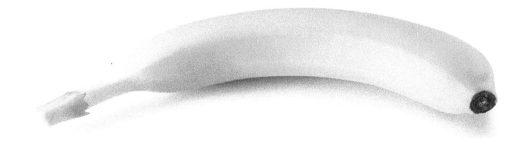

vegan dulce de leche sauce

ingredients

14-oz can unsweetened coconut milk

¾ C packed brown sugar

½ tsp coarse salt

whisk+dissolve+reduce

Whisk **one 14-oz can unsweetened coconut milk, ¾ cup packed brown sugar**, and **½ tsp coarse salt** in a heavy, large skillet on your stovetop until sugar dissolves. Increase heat to medium-high and boil until mixture is reduced to about 2½ C, stirring occasionally, about 20 minutes. Serve with pancakes!

banana dulce de leche smoothies

ingredients

2 medium frozen bananas

3 T brown sugar

pinch of salt

2 C of your favorite milk

½ tsp vanilla extract

¼ C orange juice, optional

freeze+combine

Combine **2 frozen bananas, 2 cups of your favorite milk, 3 T brown sugar, ½ tsp of vanilla extract, pinch of salt** and **¼ cup of orange juice** together into your blender.

blend+enjoy

Blend together until smooth and creamy. Enjoy!

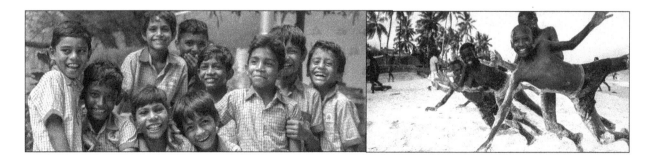

thyme for a fun activity

Salty 'Sand' Art

Ingredients:

salt
food coloring

Supplies:

clear container with lid
funnel

food-storage containers with lids
spoons.

directions

- **Pour salt into separate tupperware containers.** There's no measuring required here, just however much salt-sand you want to use!

- **Put 3-4 drops of food coloring into each container and close the lid tightly.** With your hands clasping the lid and bottom of the container, shake shake shake! (Tip: for a fun twist, play some of your favorite music and dance while you shake!)

- **After the salt is the desired color**, take off the lid and leave salt to fully dry.

- **Place your funnel into your clear container and slowly spoon in the colored salt,** one color at a time, until you get clear layers. Mix and match the layers for a beautiful design! (Tip: if you don't have a funnel, take an empty toilet paper roll and cut the length of the roll. Reroll into a cone shape.)

- **Place the lid on your container and show off your sand art!** If you make two, use them as napkin holders or small bookends. The possibilities are endless.

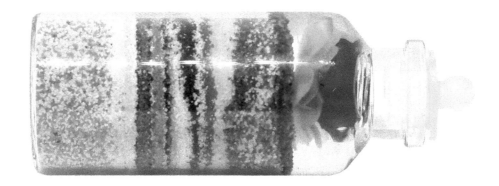

Jazzy Jamaican Jerk Butternut Squash Stew
+ Herbed Rice +
Hibiscus Tea Sparklers

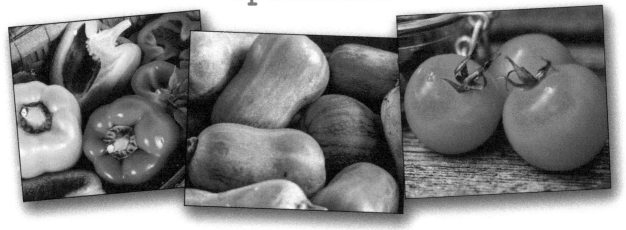

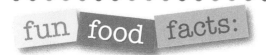

fun food facts:

Jamaican Jerk History

What exactly is "Jerk" cooking? Fragrant, savory, sweet and spicy, jerk is truly a part of Jamaica's history and can be traced back hundreds of years to the Maroons. Traditional Jamaican Jerk is a method of cooking pork. Nowadays chicken, seafood, beef, and vegetables can be seasoned in this manner as well. Jerk is a complex blend of seasonings, including scallions, onions, peppers, salt, thyme, allspice, black pepper, and many other spices. All of its ingredients grow on the island's fertile, green landscape.

During the time of slavery, the British brought slaves to Jamaica in order to guarantee a steady supply of sugar, coffee, cocoa, pimento, and other goods to merchants. A group of these slaves escaped into the mountains and were later named "the Maroons." The Maroons would blend an array of spices and herbs that they would later use to marinate and cook wild game they hunted. The meat was spiced and wrapped in leaves which helped the food keep while the Maroons were fighting the British troops. This led to the invention of the now famous "Jamaican Jerk."

Where does the word Jerk come from? According to most food history authorities, *jerk* is a Spanish word derived from the Peruvian *charqui*, or dried strips of meat similar to jerky. The word *jerk* was originally a noun, and then it later became a verb, as in "jerking," which means to poke holes in meat so the spices could be more easily permeate the meat. Jerk cooking experts say the name also could have come from either the turning of the meat in the marinade or the way some people might physically jerk a strip of meat from the roast on the grill.

The featured ingredient: Butternut Squash!

★ **Butternut squash's ancestors have been eaten for over 10,000 years.** Butternut squash originated in Mexico or Guatemala. Originally, the seeds were eaten, and the flesh of the squash was not.

★ **Butternut squash is available August through March**, though typically butternuts are at peak quality and availability in October.

★ **Although most people discard the skin and seeds of butternut squash,** the seeds are edible and quite tasty, especially if roasted and lightly salted like pumpkin seeds.

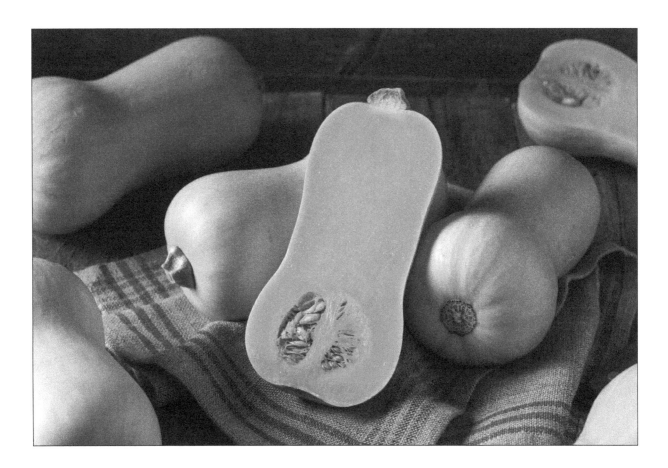

jazzy jamaican jerk butternut squash stew

ingredients

1 small bunch of green onions
1 T fresh ginger
1 clove garlic
3 T oil
1½ C canned diced tomatoes
2 T red wine vinegar
3½ tsp jerk seasoning
1 vegetable stock bouillon cube
1 package butternut squash, thawed

15-oz can black beans, rinsed and drained
1 zucchini
1 carrot
½ bell pepper
handful of fresh cilantro
salt and pepper
½ C water
2 T sugar or honey

chop+grate

Have your kids chop up **1 small bunch of green onions**, **½ bell pepper**, **1 clove of garlic**, **1 small package of frozen (thawed) butternut squash**, and **1 zucchini** into small bits. Grate **1 carrot** and **1 T fresh ginger**. Set all the vegetables to the side.

heat+fry+simmer

Heat your skillet over medium heat with **3 T of oil**. Gently add the green onion to the skillet. Soften the diced green onion in oil in your skillet for 4 minutes. Next, add the grated ginger, and **3½ tsp store bought jerk seasoning** into the skillet with the softened green onions and fry until fragrant. Stir in **1½ cups canned diced tomatoes**, the pre-chopped zucchini, **2 T red wine vinega**r, **2 T sugar or honey**, **1 vegetable stock bouillon cube**, and **½ cup water**. Bring to a simmer, cooking for 3-5 minutes, then drop in the butternut squash and simmer for 10 minutes more.

stir+simmer

Stir in **15-oz can black beans (rinsed and drained)**, bell pepper, and carrots, and simmer for at least another 5 mins until the butternut squash and carrots are tender. Have your kids mash the stew to thicken.

taste+serve

Taste before serving and add extra **salt, vinegar and/or sugar**, if needed. Add a handful of **freshly torn cilantro** on top. Serve with the rice salad and enjoy!

herbed rice salad

ingredients

2 C precooked rice (about 1 C dry)

1 T vinegar

1 T oil

1 T honey or brown sugar

½ tsp salt

½ tsp dried dill

handful fresh parsley or cilantro

precook

Precook **1 cup of dry rice** according to package directions. Set aside.

measure+whisk

Help your kids measure **1 T vinegar, 1 T oil, 1 T honey or brown sugar, ½ tsp salt** and **½ tsp of dried dill** and whisk everything up in a large salad bowl.

toss+tear+serve

Add the **2 C of precooked rice** and ask your kids to toss the rice with the dressing to combine. Allow the salad to sit for at least 30 minutes before serving so that flavors meld. Top with **handful of torn cilantro or parsley** and serve with the stew. YUM!

sparkling hibiscus ginger tea

ingredients

1-2 bags hibiscus tea

pinch freshly grated ginger

honey/sugar/stevia

3 C sparkling water

ice

steep+grate

Steep **1-2 bags of hibiscus tea** in **1 cup of hot water** for 5-7 minutes. Remove the teabag and pour the tea into a pitcher. Have your kids add **a pinch of freshly grated ginger** into the tea.

sprinkle+pour

Help your kids sprinkle some **honey or sugar or stevia** to taste (not too much) and pour in **3 C sparkling water**. Serve in cups over lots of **ice** and enjoy!

Congratulations to Young Chef Dane!
The *Global Taste Buds* Cover Star

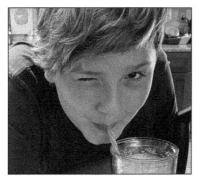

How did you first get interested in cooking?
I love cooking with my mom and it's fun for me to say I made something that people enjoy eating.

We absolutely love the connection your photo makes with an audience. How did you come up with that photo of you winking?
It's my personality to be funny and different. I was just trying the drink and it was amazing!!!

Your cookbook cover photo was taken during an online Sticky Fingers Cooking class where students prepared the Superbly Tasty Sweet 'n Sour Thai Noodle Salad + Perky Pineapple Coolers recipe. What did you enjoy about that recipe?
I liked that it was something I would have never thought I would have liked and I did like it! I especially loved the drink, and everything was healthy.

What is one of your favorite ingredients to cook with and why?
One of my favorite ingredients to use is chocolate chips because it makes everything taste way better, such as banana bread, cookies and pancakes.

Why do you think it's important for kids to get involved in the kitchen?
I think it's good for kids to cook because it gives them independence if they can make their own lunches and it gives their mom a break!

What advice would you give to young or aspiring chefs?
Cook food so you can try new things! Always take one bite, even if you don't think you'll like something.

If you could have any cooking superpower, what would it be and why?
To be able to move my hands really fast so I could chop, whisk and stir really fast!

What's a favorite food pun or joke of yours? No joke can be too 'cheesy' for us ;)
Why did the duck go into the pantry? To grab a pack of quackers!

If you could be any fruit or vegetable, what would you be and why?
I would be a kumquat because they taste terrible, so nobody would want to eat me and I would live forever!

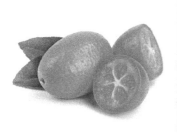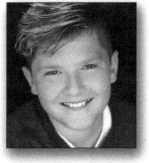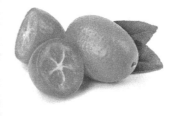

VERY GRATEFUL ACKNOWLEGMENTS

"Alone we can do so little, together we can do so much." - Helen Keller

To all of our students: Thank you for being such enthusiastic recipe testers. We couldn't have done this without all of you. Keep questioning, tasting, learning, and discovering. It's a great big, delicious world out there—keep exploring!

I truly appreciate Amy & Peregrin Marshall of Web501, Sarah Morrissey of Juniper Accounting, and Bart Writer and Randy Williams of Madison Financial who continue to support and help us lay the foundation of our Sticky Fingers Cooking journey. Snaps to Jennifer Gauerke of YellowDog Denver who designed our fun logos and helped with all of our graphics. Thank you kindly to Susan English and all of the numerous photographers (including my daughter, Ava Fletter) who all contributed to this beautiful book. Gratitude to Dane, and his parents, for submitting his wonderful photo for our cover. Deep thanks to Radha Dhruv, for all of your loving attention and kindness that you lavish on me and my family.

None of this would have been possible without my dear friend, Shannon McLaughlin. She was the first person I called when I thought a cookbook series might be a good idea. Her publishing expertise, unwavering enthusiasm, and brilliant guidance made this a much better cookbook than it might otherwise have been. That is true friendship.

A massive thank you to our phenomenal team of Chef Instructors who are undeniably the heart and soul of Sticky Fingers Cooking. We could never do what we do without your skills, care, and talents. With a special shout out to the incomparable Chef Dylan Sabuco.

To our magnificent administrative team, Katie Brennan, Kimberly Douglas, Lucy Warenski, Amanda Adams, Lauren Frontiera, Jacqui Gabel, Maggie Whittum, Chloe Sundberg, Francine Huang, Kate Bezak, Jessi Cano, Robin Pearce, Alli Doyle, Kate Bezak, Eileen Leno, and Amy Carter. Your united combination of energy, wit, compassion, creativity, attention to detail, and grit propels us forward. I'm so deeply thankful for everything you bring to the table.

A good editor will make your recipes, thoughts, ideas, and words sing. I am forever grateful to Kate Bezak, Katie Brennan, Ariel Nierenberg, Robin Pearce, Maggie Whittum, and Lucy Warenski (and her dad) for their wicked editing skills. Thank you for catching my numerous blunders and saving me from embarrassment.

Thank you to the multi-talented Francine Huang for her skillful formatting of the recipes and the book, a challenge which she tackled, no less than 9 times over, with zero complaints. Francine did let me know when she needed two weeks off to focus solely on jigsaw puzzles and coloring books in her PJ's. Many thanks to the ever artistic and effervescent, Natasha McCone, who is our lead book layout assistant. Her positive energy is always a blessing. I love to say that I have known Natasha since she was 6 months old. Because it's true.

I am fortunate enough to co-write some recipes with the abundantly talented, Jacqui Gabel. You are deliciously brilliant, Jacqui, and forever my soul sister. Thank you also to Kate Bezak who provided the wonderful activities for the book, created our index, and whose obvious love of teaching children is reflected throughout.

Laura Hall gave me the power to believe in my passion and pursue my dreams. I could only do this with your guidance, eternal love, and the endless faith you always seem to have in me. I love you, Mama.

This cookbook was creatively conceived and beautifully designed, in its entirety, by the multi-talented and ever-fascinating, Joe Hall. He co-founded Sticky Fingers Cooking with me. He works day in and day out to help build a wonderful company. He never stops creating, dreaming, and collaborating. His optimism knows no bounds. His wise kind-hearted presence is ever open and full of light. My great luck is that he is also my father. Papa, you are loved and appreciated beyond measure.

Ava, Liliana and Vivian: You are my treasures. You make me so proud. Thank you for being my beautiful, individualistic, and brilliant daughters. My tremendous love for you is immeasurable.

Finally, a world of devotion and gratefulness to my incredible husband, Ryan Fletter. A friend to all, consummate restaurateur, exciting travel companion, loving father, who also happens to be unfairly handsome. For real. Google him. Thank you, Ryan, for loving me for 25 years. Yoga pants, hare-brained ideas, cluttered kitchens, and all. Your belief in me continues to be so astonishingly absolute.

Since this is the first time I've done this, I am sure I will have unintentionally left someone out. Apologies. I am glad we have 5 more cookbooks simmering away, so I can keep fine-tuning my spoonfuls of gratitude!

Happy and Healthy Cooking,

- Erin Fletter

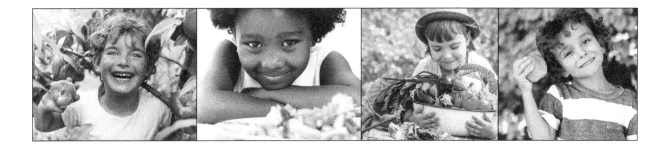

THE HANDY INDEX

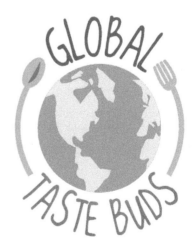

About the Author

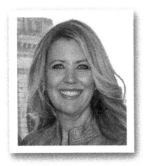

Erin Fletter

FOOD GEEK-IN-CHIEF

Erin Fletter is passionate about getting kids to not just eat, but actually crave healthy food. Erin's three enthusiastic daughters are her first round of recipe taste testers and she is never reluctant to push their culinary boundaries.

Erin loves creating hands on recipes for children that bring together fresh ingredients, global flavors, math, geography, language, nutrition, food history—and a big dash of tasty fun. Erin also writes terrible jokes about food that make everyone groan.

Erin has an extensive background in the food and wine industry and used that experience to start Sticky Fingers Cooking, a mobile and online cooking school. Sticky Fingers Cooking now has hundreds of cooking classes each week, in multiple cities and has taught over 50,000 kids how to cook. Erin lives in Denver, Colorado, with her husband, three daughters, two cats and one dog; all of whom are extremely well fed.

> "Wow, Chef Erin! You really write ALL of these recipes for Sticky Fingers? Good thing your food is a million times better than your jokes."
>
> *- Avery, age 6*

CPSIA information can be obtained
at www.ICGtesting.com
Printed in the USA
BVHW020210280521
608367BV00017B/506

9 781637 322246